Public Health: Practices, Methods and Policies

Joav Merrick (Series Editor)
Division for Intellectual and Developmental Disabilities, Ministry of Social Affairs and Social Services, Jerusalem, Israel

"Public Health" is a book series with publications from a multidisciplinary group of researchers, practitioners and clinicians for an international professional forum interested in the broad spectrum of public health issues.

About the Editor-in-Chief
Joav Merrick, MD, MMedSci, DMSc, born and educated in Denmark is Professor of Pediatrics affiliated with the Division of Pediatrics, Hadassah Hebrew University Medical Center, Mt Scopus Campus, Jerusalem, Israel, Kentucky Children's Hospital, University of Kentucky, Lexington, United States and Professor of Public Health at the Center for Healthy Development, School of Public Health, Georgia State University, Atlanta, United States, the former medical director of the Disability Administration, Ministry of Social Affairs and Social Services, Jerusalem and the founder and director of the National Institute of Child Health and Human Development in Israel. Email: jmerrick@zahav.net.il

nova
Medicine & Health
New York

Public Health: Practices, Methods and Policies

Public Health: Recent International Research
Joav Merrick, MD, MMedSci, DMSc (Editor), Mohammed Morad, MD (Editor)
2022. ISBN: 978-1-68507-491-3 (Hardcover)
2022. ISBN: 978-1-68507-638-2 (eBook)

Environmental Justice and the Intersection of Poverty, Racism and Child Health Disparities
I. Leslie Rubin, MD (Editor), Joav Merrick, MD, MMedSci, DMSc (Editor)
2022. ISBN: 978-1-68507-489-0 (Hardcover)
2022. ISBN: 978-1-68507-640-5 (eBook)

Science, Culture, and Politics: Despair and Hope in the Time of a Pandemic
Consolato M. Sergi, MD (Author)
2021. ISBN: 978-1-53619-816-4 (Hardcover)
2021. ISBN: 978-1-68507-161-5 (eBook)

The COVID-19 Pandemic: A Tribute to the Corona Whistleblowers
Søren Ventegodt, MD
Niels Jørgen Andersen, MSc
Joav Merrick, MD, MMedSci, DMSc,
2020. ISBN: 978-1-53618-146-3 (Hardcover)
2020. ISBN: 978-1-53618-236-1 (eBook)

Public Health Themes in Grenada and the Caribbean Region
Joav Merrick, MD, MMedSci, DMSc, (Editor)
Lindonne Glasgow, MSPH, DrPH (Editor)
2020. ISBN: 978-1-53618-118-0 (Hardcover)
2020. ISBN: 978-1-53618-119-7 (eBook)

More information about this series can be found at
https://novapublishers.com/product-category/series/public-health-practices-methods-and-policies/

I Leslie Rubin and Joav Merrick
Editors

Environmental Health

Poverty, Race and Child Health in the Time of COVID-19

nova
Medicine & Health
New York

https://doi.org/10.52305/NIQR1132

Library of Congress Cataloging-in-Publication Data

ISBN: 979-8-88697-292-4

Published by Nova Science Publishers, Inc. † New York

Contents

Introduction

Chapter 1

Intersection of poverty, race and child health in the time of COVID-19: 16th annual *Break the Cycle* of children's environmental health disparities program and student projects

I Leslie Rubin[1-5,*], MD, Abby Mutic[3,4,8], APRN, PhD, Claire D Coles[3,11,12], PhD, Victoria Green[3,7], JD MD, Rebecca Philipsborn[2,3], MD, MPA, Melissa Gittinger[3,6], DO, Nathan Mutic[3,4,8], Wayne Garfinkel[3,10], BSCE, Henry Falk[3], MD, MPH, Benjamin A Gitterman[9], MD and Joav Merrick[13-17], MD, MMedSci, DMSc

[1]Department of Pediatrics, Morehouse School of Medicine, Atlanta, Georgia
[2]Department of Pediatrics, Emory University School of Medicine, Atlanta, Georgia, United States of America
[3]Southeast Pediatric Environmental Health Specialty Unit, Emory University, Atlanta, Georgia, United States of America
[4]Break the Cycle of Health Disparities, Inc. Atlanta, Georgia, United States of America
[5]The Rubin Center for Autism and Developmental Pediatrics, Atlanta, Georgia, United States of America
[6]Georgia Poison Center, Grady Health System, Atlanta, Georgia, United States of America

* *Correspondence:* I Leslie Rubin, MD, Associate Professor, Department of Pediatrics, Morehouse School of Medicine, Director, Break the Cycle Program of the Southeast Pediatric Environmental Health Specialty Unit at Emory University, Founder, Break the Cycle of Health Disparities Inc, Medical Director, The Rubin Center for Autism and Developmental Pediatrics. 750 Hammond Drive, Building 1, Suite 100, Atlanta, GA 30328, United States. Email: lrubi01@emory.edu.

In: Environmental Health
Editors: I Leslie Rubin and Joav Merrick
ISBN: 979-8-88697-292-4

[7]Department of Gynecology and Obstetrics, Emory University School of Medicine, Atlanta, Georgia, United States of America
[8]Nell Hodgson Woodruff School of Nursing, Emory University, Atlanta, Georgia, United States of America
[9]Departments of Pediatrics and Public Health, George Washington University Schools of Medicine and Public Health and Health Services, General and Community Pediatrics, Children's National Medical Center, Washington DC, United States of America
[10]Retired EPA Region 4 Children's Environmental Health Coordinator, Atlanta, Georgia,
[11]MotherToBaby, Atlanta, Georgia, United States of America
[12]Department of Psychiatry and Behavioral Sciences and Pediatrics, Emory University School of Medicine, Atlanta, Georgia, , United States of America
[13]National Institute of Child Health and Human Development, Jerusalem, Israel
[14]Office of the Medical Director, Health Services, Division for Intellectual and Developmental Disabilities, Ministry of Social Affairs and Social Services, Jerusalem, Israel
[15]Division of Pediatrics, Hadassah Hebrew University Medical Center, Mt Scopus Campus, Jerusalem, Israel
[16]Kentucky Children's Hospital, University of Kentucky College of Medicine, Lexington, Kentucky, United States of America
[17]Center for Human Development, School of Public Health, Georgia State University, Atlanta, Georgia, United States of America

Abstract

Break the Cycle of Children's Environmental Health Disparities (*Break the Cycle*) is an annual collaborative interdisciplinary research and training program involving university students in academic tracks focusing on the impact of adverse social, economic, and environmental factors on children's health, development, education, and prospects for their future. The target populations are communities where there is a substantial measure of poverty associated with social, ethnic, racial, and political marginalization, an increased likelihood of environmental exposures, and environmental injustice with high risks for adverse impacts on children's health and well-being. Participating students are required to develop projects that focus on preventing or reducing adverse environmental factors or their impact on children's health, and promote positive practices to improve the future outcome for children who live in these communities. Student projects cover a wide range of adverse social and environmental factors and their associated intergenerational health implications across the lifespan, and propose solutions at an individual, family, community, and societal level, with the potential for a positive outcome. At the end of the project period, participating students are required to present the results of their work at a national conference and then write a manuscript for publication. The chapters in this book represent the work of students who participated in the 16th Annual *Break the Cycle* program 2020-2021. The phrase *Break the Cycle* in this context uses the ecological construct of the cycle of environmental health disparities and offers a framework for tackling health disparities and promoting health equity among children who are vulnerable as a consequence of adverse social, economic, environmental and political factors.

Introduction

Children are more vulnerable to environmental exposures than adults. Children breathe more air, drink more water and eat more food for their body weight than adults, so their potential chemical exposure load through polluted air, water and soil is greater. Furthermore, their organs and organ systems as well as physiologic and metabolic processes are still in development, so they are more vulnerable to immediate and long-term negative health outcomes of adverse environmental factors (1). Children who grow up in circumstances of poverty are likely to live in areas where they are exposed to a greater pollution load and are more likely to experience physiological and psychological stresses with financial, educational, housing and food insecurity. The combination of social and emotional stresses with the added exposure to environmental toxins, cumulatively affect their health, education, and potential for success in society (2, 3).

Children from poor families live in poor neighborhoods where housing tends to be older and therefore more likely to have residual lead paint. Children who live in these older houses are more likely to be exposed to lead and therefore, to have high blood lead levels (4). Lead is a neurotoxin that causes brain damage resulting in cognitive impairment, with learning difficulties, attention deficit hyperactivity disorder (ADHD) and behavior problems including aggression (5, 6). These factors adversely affect children's ability to function optimally in school, making it less likely for them to graduate which compromises their earning potential and keeps them in poverty. Furthermore, the schools in poor neighborhoods tend to be poorly funded because funding support for schools is partially dependent on property taxes, which, in poor communities are low (7). So, it follows, poor neighborhoods have low-income families, therefore, the tax revenue is low and consequently the funding for the school is low. This disparity in funding for schools affects the state of repair of the buildings and the quality of the indoor environment in the buildings, as well as the salaries of the teachers and staff and the quality of education (8, 9). The cumulative impact of poverty, lead exposure, and poor education, results in lower academic scores, with a greater likelihood for children to fail grades, drop out of school and thereafter, struggle for meaningful employment and income (10, 11).

Children who live poorer urban neighborhoods are also more likely to live near roadways where the air is more heavily polluted with exhaust from motor vehicles, increasing the risks for asthma. Also, older houses in these neighborhoods are more likely to have malfunctioning heating and air ventilation systems, resulting in the growth of mold, especially in wetter climates. The presence of mold correlates with a higher likelihood of allergies and asthma and associated adverse consequences on health, including emergency room visits for acute episodes of reactive airway disease with a greater likelihood of absences from school and more hospitalizations with increased mortality (6, 12, 13).

Poor neighborhoods are also more likely to be situated near factories or other sources of pollution with toxic waste, which results in poor air quality and contaminated water and soil. These conditions, taken together, impact poor children and their families disproportionately and cumulatively (10). The placement of factories and polluting industries near poor neighborhoods putting affected communities at risk for a variety of adverse health outcomes, constitutes environmental injustice (14, 15).

Thus, children who grow up in poverty are more likely to be exposed to multiple adverse physical, chemical, and social elements in their environment and are more likely to be emotionally stressed, with multiple elements of insecurity with anxiety and fear (16). The combination of emotional and environmental stresses takes a toll on the physiological, neurological, immunological, educational, and psychological well-being of children leaving them with metabolic and hemodynamic consequences on their cardiovascular, immune, and endocrine systems, resulting in an increased likelihood of adverse health outcomes in adulthood including obesity, diabetes, and hypertension (17).

Furthermore, the neighborhood environment in poor areas, with crowded houses, greater likelihood of vehicular traffic, poor lighting, and likely presence of trash, provide the dystopian setting for drug dealing, crime, and violence, with little to no green spaces and suitable facilities for recreation (6, 18). These conditions also increase the risks of crime with fear of assault, a greater likelihood of being exposed to street drugs and drug dealers, and increased likelihood of gun violence (19).

As children reach adolescence, they are more likely to experience school failure and engage in risky behavior, including substance abuse, gang membership, and crime. Many of these young people drop out of school and face limited employment options. As a consequence, they are more likely to carry a relatively dim view of their future, and may resort to drugs to feel better or crime to make money to survive or support their habits or lifestyles. These behaviors can result in incarceration, or in the most extreme instances death from drugs or gun violence, with the emotional and social consequences for the individual, the family, the community and society (20). This scenario plays out in too many cities and states in the US, which has the highest incarceration rate in the world with a disproportionate percentage of young men of color in prison (21). It is noteworthy, and reason for a modicum of optimism, that, since its peak in the 1990s with over 100,000 children in prison, the number of juvenile justice cases has decreased substantially, but remains at a disturbing 36,000 with more than 500 children under 12 years of age in 2019 (22). Although this positive trend is a result of local, state, and federal processes, making positive change in the lives of vulnerable children, it begins with taking individual action and striving to make a positive difference in the lives of vulnerable children, not only in reducing the negative environmental factors, but in promoting resilience through education with strong emotional and social support (23).

In summary, these adverse environmental and emotional stresses, along with negative educational experiences, compromise learning, and correlate with high drop-out rates and low graduation rates (24). Limited education leads to poor employment opportunities, or work with low pay, trapping young people in the poorer neighborhoods with older houses in states of disrepair, contributing to exposures to indoor hazards of lead, mold, and other possible contaminants, as well as higher rates of mental health disorders such as depression, anxiety about the future, despair, and social isolation (25). The assault of adverse social, economic, and environmental factors on vulnerable children results in unfavorable health, developmental, and educational outcomes and compromises a child's opportunity for economic and social success in life. This persistent pattern devolves into the perpetuation of an intergenerational cycle, the codification of which, can be represented in an ecological construct that embodies the concept of the cycle of children's environmental health disparities (see Figure 1) (26).

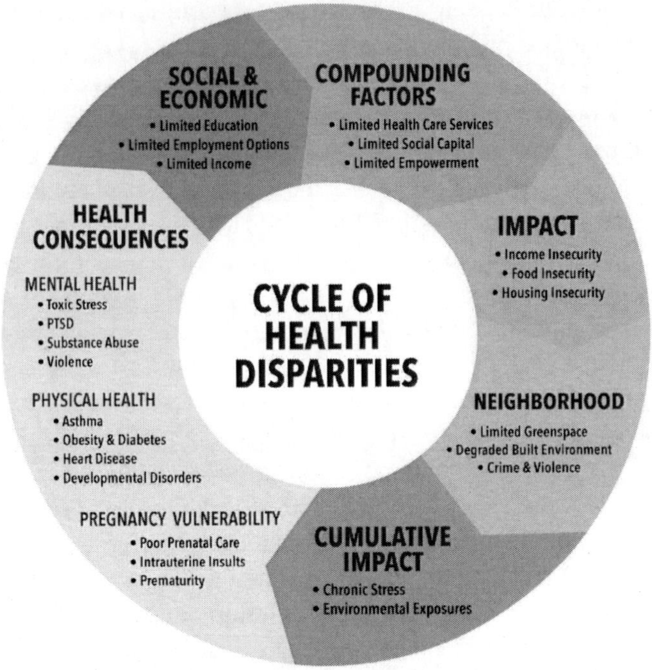

Figure 1. Cycle of environmental health disparities (26).

Intersection of poverty, race and child health in the United States

The profile for children in poverty is that their parents tend to have lower educational attainment and are less likely to be employed. Furthermore, the children are more likely to live in a single parent household, most often a single mother, or, at times, a grandmother (27). Children from single parent households are four times more likely to be poor compared to children in two-parent families (27). What these statistics do not tell us is that children who are poor are disproportionately represented by children of color. The Children's Defense Fund reports that approximately 1 in 3 African American children, 1 in 3 Native American children and nearly 1 in 4 Hispanic American children were living in poverty compared with 1 in 11 white children, and that almost two-thirds of Black, Hispanic, and Native American children live in areas of concentrated poverty, compared with one-third of white children (28). If one then correlates racial and ethnic status with health, using infant mortality as a proxy, the infant mortality rate is more than double in the Black (10.8) and almost double in Native American (8.2) populations compared to the White population (4.6) (29).

The centuries-long history of slavery and continued political and economic oppression and suppression of people of color, whether they be of African descent, of Native American descent or from other parts of the world such as Latin America, has resulted in the concentration of poverty in communities of color across the US (15). There are clear political and economic factors that continue to play a significant role in creating the disproportionate environmental impacts on the affected individuals, communities, and populations (30). Discrimination and bias leveled at groups of people is racism, which expresses itself at many levels of society, from the individual interaction, through provision of services, such as healthcare and education, to employment, career advancement, social status, and all manner of social and economic life (31). The impact of racism on health disparities exacerbates and aggravates the impact of poverty. This phenomenon has led the CDC to declare that racism is a prominent cause of health inequities and a threat to public health (32). The American Academy of Pediatrics identifies racism as a core social determinant of health linked to birth disparities, adverse physical and mental health problems in children and adolescents (33). Furthermore, the ongoing health problems continue to plague the children as they grow into adulthood, increasing the health burden with chronic diseases, further reducing employment opportunities and earning potential, reducing life expectancy and adding cumulative costs to society (33).

COVID-19 pandemic and children's health disparities

In the early days of the COVID-19 pandemic, it became clear that there were groups of people who were more vulnerable to the infection, more likely to be sick enough to require hospitalization, and were also more likely to die from the severe complications of the infection. It also became clear that older individuals and individuals with preexisting respiratory, cardiac, or metabolic disorders, such as obesity and diabetes, were more susceptible and more likely to succumb to the disease (34). Over the course of the COVID-19 Pandemic, what has become abundantly clear, however, is that people from low-income and minority neighborhoods are much more susceptible to contracting the virus and more likely to get sick enough to require hospitalization and more likely to die from the disease in disproportionately large numbers (35). Identifiers such as poverty, overcrowding, congregate living, crowded workplaces, and lack of protective measures, mark these vulnerable populations as being at increased risk (36, 37). These are the same populations who have an increased burden of disease by virtue of their social, economic, and environmental vulnerability and are the focus of the *Break the Cycle* program. What the COVID-19 pandemic effectively revealed, was that the vulnerability of disadvantaged populations to adverse health conditions is predictable (38).

Now, two years after the initial rude awakening and response to the global impact of COVID-19, particularly the susceptibility seen in vulnerable populations at a local and national level, we have also seen glaring disparities globally, between the more affluent countries and the low resource countries. The practical realities are that affluent people could escape behind barriers with all the comforts in their isolation, while the poorer people had to endure the daily struggles for survival, to secure food for their families and, at the same time, face the ubiquitous and deadly virus in crowded and unprotected circumstances. It is no wonder that the disparities in morbidity and mortality were great in local, national, and international communities and societies (39, 40).

From the outset, children were less likely to become infected and had less severe symptoms (34). At the time of writing, the American Academy of Pediatrics reported that the infection rate for children is less than 20% of cumulative cases with less than 5% of hospitalizations and less than 0.3% of all deaths (41). Although children did not get the infection to the same degree as adults, children did succumb to an aggressive form of the infection, affecting multiple organ systems. This Multisystem Inflammatory Disease (MIS-C) affected 1 in 3,000-4,000 children who had COVID-19, but it also exhibited disparities in prevalence and impact (42). Compared with the general population, MIS-C was more frequent among non-Hispanic Black children (183% of expected) and Hispanic children (139%) than among non-Hispanic White children (64%) and non-Hispanic Asian children (48%). Compared with children with COVID-19, MIS-C was more frequent in non-Hispanic Black children (207% of expected) as well as among Hispanic (102%) and less frequent in non-Hispanic Asian (74%) non-Hispanic White children (68%) (43).

Despite the lower rate of infection with COVID-19 and the relatively mild expression of the disease in children, and even the rare but dramatic presentations of MIS-C, children suffered in many more ways, less physical than psychological, emotional, and social. During the early period of lockdown, children were restricted in their ability to exercise their natural need for physical activity and socialization, as well as meet their need for a good education to help them succeed in life. Here too, children from low-income families, communities and societies tended to suffer more because of the crowded home situations, inadequate ventilation, poor indoor air quality, limited resources, lack of greenspace, and lack of internet access to avail themselves of the opportunity for remote learning. Overall, the psychological, emotional, educational, and social impact was, and remains great, particularly for low-income families and communities who are also marginalized for one reason or another (44).

One of the biggest impacts of the COVID-19 pandemic on children has been the death of family members, particularly parents and other caregivers. From April 1, 2020 through June 30, 2021, an estimated 140,000 children under age 18 in the United States lost a parent, custodial grandparent, or grandparent caregiver who provided the child's home and basic needs, including love, security, and daily care (45) That translates into approximately 1 out of 500 children in the United States who has experienced COVID-19-associated orphanhood or death of a grandparent caregiver, with children from racial and ethnic minority groups accounting for 65% of those who lost a primary caregiver due to the pandemic, while representing on 35% of the population (45).

When looking at the loss of primary and secondary caregivers to COVID-19 by race/ethnicity, the statistics varied dramatically: 1 of every 168 American Indian/Alaska Native children, 1 of every 310 Black children, 1 of every 412 Hispanic children, 1 of every 612 Asian children, and 1 of every 753 White children experienced orphanhood or death of caregivers. Thus, compared to white children, American Indian/Alaska Native children were 4.5 times more likely to lose a parent or grandparent caregiver, Black children were 2.4 times more likely, and Hispanic children were nearly 2 times (1.8) more likely (46).

Children's lives are permanently changed by the loss of a mother, father, or grandparent who provided a home, with basic needs, and loving care, with significant adverse long-term consequences, such as mental health problems (45). This is particularly acute and devastating in single parent families (27). With the loss of an anchor in life, children can suffer more serious consequences such as engaging in risky social behaviors that could lead to substance abuse, sexual activity, and violence as well as being vulnerable to physical emotional and sexual abuse, and exploitation, which can lead to an increased risk of suicide (45).

Climate change, environmental justice and children's health disparities

Climate change represents an inescapable and inexorable cumulative and compounding factor in addressing children's environmental health disparities. Just as the COVID-19 pandemic revealed the dramatic disparities in its impact on children born into poverty and into marginalized families and communities of color, so too does the impact of climate change.

According to NOAA, Earth's temperature has risen by 0.14°F (0.08°C) per decade since 1880, and the rate of warming over the past 40 years is more than twice that: 0.32°F (0.18°C) per decade since 1981, and 2020 was the second-warmest year on record (47).

Extreme heat affects all children, especially infants who are most vulnerable to dehydration from the heat, and teenagers who engage in strenuous outdoor sport (48, 49). Children in low-income and under-resourced communities are more vulnerable because they live in neighborhoods where they are less likely to have green spaces with parks and trees to provide relief, resulting in a 'heat island' in urban areas with temperatures about 1–7°F higher than temperatures in outlying areas and nighttime temperatures about 2–5°F higher (50). Thus, children living in the same city can experience vastly different ambient temperatures in any heat event, and that children in low-income and racially diverse blocks of the neighborhood will experience more heat, compounded by limited resources to escape from the heat (51).

Moreover, with the increase in global temperatures, there are more perturbations in the climate resulting in an increased number and intensity of natural disasters, such as hurricanes, floods, wildfires and other extreme weather events, which wreak havoc on the natural environment, the built environment, and the people living in and near the event. The impact of these disasters is both costly to society and can be devastating to the communities and families in their path and in their wake (52). Here again, it is the children who are most vulnerable especially those living in the most socially, economically, racially, and geographically vulnerable areas (53, 54). These children not only experience the direct impact of the disaster with higher rates of morbidity and mortality, but also suffer long-term from the traumatic experience, from the loss of everything they have known, from the loss of family members, and from the dislocation and struggle to settle into unfamiliar and maybe even hostile places. These adverse experiences can result in significant mental health problems, affecting their learning and education, that can last a lifetime (55).

Thus, children from poor and minority communities, who are predominantly children of color, are most vulnerable to environmental hazards and to the rapidly growing forces of climate change. The cumulative environmental impact of adverse social, economic, physical, chemical, and psychological exposures has a more powerful effect on children at the intersection of poverty, racism, and climate change.

Conclusion

Poverty and racism become inseparable in the formulations of children's health disparities, and the urban and rural landscapes compounded by environmental injustice, become the great interdisciplinary challenge for our society. These factors are tested by the powerful and unpredictable local, national and global disasters such as we have experienced with the COVID-19 pandemic and the existential threat of climate change with its associated extreme weather events. To this end, our *Break the Cycle* program invites students to develop projects from many different perspectives, from the molecular chemical toxin to the physical health and wellbeing, to the social and emotional stresses, to the legal, ethical, and political struggles, to reduce health disparities and promote health equity for all children. It is anticipated that the results of the projects will make a difference, individually and cumulatively, and that each of the students who participate in the program will go on to leadership roles in making a positive difference in the world, especially for the most vulnerable children.

Break the Cycle program

Break the Cycle is an annual, collaborative interdisciplinary research and training program involving university students in academic tracks that focus on the impact of adverse social, economic, and environmental factors on children's health, development, and education. Each participating university student develops a project that focuses on preventing or reducing environment-related disorders for children who live in communities where the cumulative impact of environmental hazards and emotional stresses are related to circumstances of social, economic, or racial disadvantage. At the conclusion of the project period, the students present the results of their projects at a national conference and write manuscripts on their projects for publication in a peer-reviewed journal supplement dedicated to the collection of projects from each annual program as well as in this book.

The annual program begins with a call for proposals from a wide range of university students. Proposals are evaluated by a competitive review process for the quality of the proposal, its relevance to children's environmental health disparities, creativity, and feasibility. Ten students are selected to work with their academic mentors and their home universities, and with *Break the Cycle* faculty, to complete their projects. The students and their mentors are required to participate in monthly conference calls, during which the progress of each project is reviewed, additional perspectives are explored, and constructive guidance is provided. During these conference calls, students and their mentors also have an opportunity to communicate and collaborate with their counterparts at other universities.

Fundamental to *Break the Cycle* is the expectation that the projects make a positive difference by improving the health and well-being of children, their families, and their communities. It is also envisioned that the students would be inspired to pursue careers that focus on reducing health disparities and in becoming leaders for the future. Furthermore, because each student is required to have a mentor at their home university, it is anticipated that the faculty mentors add to the literature and body of science on the subject into their curricula, and thereby promote further research and academic interest in this field (see Table 1).

It is also anticipated that participating students inspire peers in their academic, professional, and social circles, and that the interdisciplinary nature of the program with participation of students at other universities around the world be stimulating and inspiring (Table 2). A 2012 survey of alumni of the program demonstrated that students derive significant benefit from all aspects of their participation in the process, which include the practical aspects of conducting a research project, in preparing and delivering a presentation, and in writing a manuscript. The manuscripts which are published in this volume, provide for the students an asset for further academic or employment opportunities. Each student gains knowledge about children's environmental health and environmental health disparities as well as being exposed to different perspectives from the other student projects. Many participants report that their participation in the program influenced their career choice (56).

Table 1. Project guidelines

• University faculty identify students who have an interest in this topic area and support the student in the selection of ideas for projects that explore environmental factors that adversely affect the health of children living in circumstances of social and economic disadvantage. Alternatively, students interested in a specific project can initiate the application process and identify mentors to work with them.
• The students submit their proposals which are reviewed by the *Break the Cycle* faculty. The process is competitive with only 10 projects being selected each year.
• During the project period, there are monthly conference calls with all students and mentors to monitor the progress of their projects, share ideas, and assure that the projects are consistent with the spirit of the *Break the Cycle* concept.
• At the end of the project period, the students present the results of their work at the annual *Break the Cycle* conference.
• The students are then required to write papers on their projects, which are submitted for publication in an international journal as a monograph of the *Break the Cycle* projects. The papers are also published as chapters in a book as part of a public health series.
• The progress and careers of the participating students are tracked to evaluate the impact of their participation in the *Break the Cycle* program.

Table 2. Desired outcomes

• To inspire students from a variety of academic disciplines to explore the impact of adverse social, economic, environmental, and political factors on the health, development, and education of children, and to creatively generate strategies to address the challenges.
• To collaborate with an interdisciplinary team of academic leaders from a variety of different universities and colleges to get a perspective on the broader issues of this topic area.
• To encourage faculty at universities who participate in this program to promote academic interest and social awareness in children's environmental health disparities.
• To cultivate future leaders among the students

Since its inception in 2004, *Break the Cycle* has held 15 annual programs and worked with over 150 students representing 50 different university departments in 12 states in the US, as well as students from countries in Latin America, Europe, and Africa. To date, 13 monographs have been published in international journals and 13 books in a public health series. In the 2012 survey, alumni rated their experience with Break the Cycle as valuable, with many reporting that they pursued careers relating to their *Break the Cycle* projects (56).

Break the Cycle 16 projects

The papers in this publication represent the interdisciplinary array of creative work by students from universities in the US as well as from South Africa who participated in the 16th Annual *Break the Cycle* program in 2020. As usual, the papers in this volume cover a wide range of topic areas including the critical importance of toxic chemicals, nutrition and neighborhoods, greenspaces, COVID-19 and coping with the loss of a parent. The following are the abstracts for the *Break the Cycle* 16 student projects found in this volume:

Student papers

An examination of the prevalence of COVID-19 in the Texas Juvenile Justice System

Trainee: Rachel J Slover; Mentor: Rebecca Fry; Institution: University of North Carolina, Chapel Hill, NC

Abstract: COVID-19 has posed a nationwide public health emergency, and one of the most at-risk yet concurrently overlooked populations in the United States has been youth in the juvenile justice system. In order to understand how to break the cycle of environmental health disparities faced by incarcerated youth, an examination was performed of the prevalence of COVID-19 in the juvenile justice system through a Texas case study – chosen due to the state's large incarcerated youth population, vulnerability to COVID-19, and transparency in data reporting. Data on demographics and COVID-19 case counts were gathered on Texas Juvenile Justice Department (TJJD) facilities to understand who comprises the at-risk population and the extent of that risk. The potential for community influence on facility vulnerability was examined through data from the NIEHS Pandemic Vulnerability Index (PVI) and data from the TJJD on staff COVID-19 case counts. Analysis found racial disparities between placement in high versus lower-security TJJD facilities and between the state and TJJD population compositions. Findings further demonstrated baseline TJJD county vulnerability, high COVID-19 case counts for incarcerated youth, likely disease vectors from the staff to the youth, and disparities in case counts between facilities. Further research should be conducted to assess the sources of the disparities and how to best inform methods to break the cycle of health disparities and strive for equitable youth justice.

Six month outcomes of malnourished children enrolled in the nutritional therapeutic program in a peri-urban, low-income settlement in the Western Cape, South Africa

Trainee: Suzanne Kerswill; Mentor: Etienne Nel; Institution: University of Stellenbosch, Cape Town, South Africa

Abstract: Childhood malnutrition continues to be a major challenge in South Africa, contributing to almost a third of deaths under the age of five, and the prevalence of under-five growth stunting has remained static at around 27% since 1999. The success of Community-based Therapeutic Care (CTC) in reducing mortality from severe acute malnutrition is well documented, although the sustainability of short-term successes is unknown. Modelled on CTC principles, the Nutrition Therapeutic Program (NTP) has been well established in the Western Cape in South Africa, but outcomes of this six-month program have yet to be measured. The aim of our study is to determine outcomes of malnourished children after 6 months on the NTP, looking at weight gain, defaulting rates, and mortality, and to compare these outcomes to international Sphere standards. A retrospective descriptive cohort study was conducted in a peri-urban, low-income settlement in the Western Cape. 270 patients meeting criteria for malnutrition between the age of 6 months and 5 years were recruited from 3 community clinics between January 2017-December 2018. Outcomes revealed a mortality rate of 0,7%, which was below the international Sphere target of <3%. Other outcomes did not meet Sphere targets, with a defaulting rate of 53% (target <15%), success rate of 27% (target >75%), and average daily weight gain at 6 months of 0,76g/kg/day (target >3g/kg/day). We concluded that Sphere targets may not be appropriate success metrics in this context, as the increased length of the program may be responsible for the higher defaulting rates, whilst recourse to in-hospital treatment means lower mortality rates are achievable. We feel that clear, achievable, and tailored local targets should be set to motivate healthcare practitioners to address the problem of childhood malnutrition in South Africa.

Does early life phthalate exposure mediate racial disparities in children's cognitive abilities?

Trainee: Marisa A Patti; Mentor: Joseph M Braun; Institution: Brown University, Providence, RI

Abstract: Exposure to phthalates is associated with diminished cognition. It is unknown, however, if disproportionate exposure to phthalates among racial minorities contributes to racial disparities in children's intellectual abilities. Methods: We used data from 253 mother-child pairs in Cincinnati, OH (HOME Study, 2003-2006). We measured urinary concentrations of eleven phthalate metabolites twice during pregnancy and up to six times in childhood. We evaluated children's cognitive abilities at ages 5 and 8 years. Using causal mediation models, we quantified covariate-adjusted direct and indirect effects of race on children's Full Scale IQ scores for individual phthalate metabolite concentrations during gestation and childhood. Results: Average IQ scores among Black children (n = 90) were 7.0-points lower (95% CI: -12, -1.8) than White children (n = 145) after adjustment for socioeconomic factors. Urinary monobenzyl phthalate (MBzP) and monoethyl phthalate (MEP) concentrations during gestation and childhood were higher among Black children. We did not observe compelling evidence that phthalate mediated the race-IQ association, with the exception of MEP. Childhood MEP concentrations partially mediated the race-IQ association. For instance, the disparities in IQ scores between Black and White children would have been reduced by 1.9 points (95% CI: -4.7, 0.7) for each 10-fold reduction in urinary MEP concentrations at age 2 years. Other phthalate metabolite concentrations during pregnancy or childhood did not mediate the race-IQ association. Conclusions: We found that urinary MEP concentrations partly mediated IQ disparities among HOME Study children. Reducing exposure to some phthalates might help reduce IQ disparities among Black and White children.

Phthalate exposure in children: Assessing knowledge, attitudes and behaviors in families with low socioeconomic status

Trainee: Rachana Charla; Mentor: David Collier; Institution: East Carolina University, Greenville, NC

Abstract: Phthalates are a family of synthetic chemicals used in the manufacturing of plastic products, scented products, and personal care products. Exposure to phthalates is a concern as they are considered endocrine disrupting chemicals (EDCs). Here we employed a survey to assess the knowledge, attitudes, and behaviors (KAB) related to phthalates and the use of personal care products that may contain phthalates among 50 parents and caregivers with children no more than five years old at the Brody School of Medicine's Pediatric Outpatient Clinic found at East Carolina University. We found significant relationships between race and product usage with Black respondents more likely to use spray air fresheners, lotions, and candles compared to the non-Black respondents. Additionally, there were significant correlations between income and education level regarding knowledge and recognition of terms like phthalates. Low socioeconomic status (SES) and lack of knowledge notably affect potential phthalate exposure in children from personal care products as well as cleaning products. Further studies are needed to confirm the significance of these observations.

Comparison of neighborhood deprivation index and food desert status as environmental predictors of early childhood obesity

Trainee: Shannon C Conrey; Mentor: Ardythe L Morrow; Institution: University of Cincinnati, Cincinnati, OH

Abstract: Nearly 14% of American children aged 2–5 have obesity, with higher rates in children from lower-income and Black families. While evidence connects neighborhood socio-economic environment (SEE) and obesity in adults and adolescents, little is known of this relationship in young children. We compared measures of SEE and family-level socio-demographic factors as predictors of obesity at age two. Methods: Family-level data from the PREVAIL Cohort, a CDC-funded birth cohort in Cincinnati, Ohio, were collected prenatally from the mothers. Residential addresses were geocoded and assigned validated measures of census tract-level SEE, including USDA food desert indicators and the Deprivation Index. Family-level and ecological SEE were compared as predictors of obesity (BMIz $\geq$ 1.65) at age two in terms of proportional differences, relative risk, and model fit statistics. Results: Residing outside of Deprivation Index High SEE neighborhoods was significantly associated with higher proportion (20.0% *vs* 5.9%; $\chi^2 = 4.36$, $p = 0.037$) and increased risk of obesity in univariable (RR = 3.4, 95%CI: 1.26–13.86) and multivariable models (RR = 3.5, 95%CI: 1.06–11.71). There were no differences in proportion or risk of obesity by USDA food desert indicators or family-level factors. Models using categorical Deprivation Index performed better than the family-level and the USDA food desert variables in terms of model fit. Conclusion: In the PREVAIL Cohort, only category of Deprivation Index was a significant predictor of obesity in two-year-old children. Future studies are needed to evaluate the Deprivation Index as a generalizable tool to identify neighborhoods at higher risk for obesity.

Investigating equitable access to greenspace during the COVID-19 pandemic: Implications for children's mental health in Durham, North Carolina

Trainee: Sharmi Amin; Mentors: Kate Hoffman, Catherine Kastleman, Heather M Stapleton; Institution: Duke University, Durham, NC

Abstract: Past research suggests positive correlations between time spent outdoors and better mental health in children. During the COVID-19 pandemic, researchers predicted that limitations on social gathering could have lasting impacts on children's mental well-being. We hypothesized that protective guidelines set in place to prevent COVID-19 infection would decrease children's time spent in greenspaces, adversely impacting mental well-being. We also investigated changes in children's time spent outdoors during the pandemic, the social and structural barriers to accessing local greenspaces, and the potential impacts on children's mental health in Durham, North Carolina, USA. An online survey was distributed via parent Facebook groups to collect data (n = 95 children). The Pediatric Symptom Checklist (PSC) was used as a proxy for indicating children's mental well-being. Most parents indicated a change in the amount of time spent outside during the pandemic. Children who spent more time outdoors in general, and children who spent more time outdoors during the pandemic, had lower PSC scores, indicating better mental well-being. When examining barriers to greenspace access, we observed no difference in the walkability index between higher- and lower-income zip codes. We did find that those residing in lower-income zip codes indicated more safety concerns about greenspaces particularly related to criminal activity. However, we found that the distribution of PSC scores was lower for children living in lower-income zip codes compared to higher-income zip codes, suggesting better mental well-being. Cumulatively, our results indicate that time spent outdoors has positive impacts on children's mental health.

Neighborhood quality and positive health indicators among urban adolescents

Trainee: Han N Oo; Mentor: Julie B Herbstman; Institution: Columbia University, New York, NY

Abstract: There is a growing epidemiologic interest to expand the scope of health research beyond disease and risk factors to a more comprehensive evaluation of all health states, including those on the positive end of the spectrum ("positive health"). Neighborhood quality (NQ) is a potentially modifiable factor that may influence positive health. We evaluated the association between perception of NQ in childhood and indicators of positive health among adolescents who live in low-income, urban neighborhoods of New York City. Mothers assessed NQ prospectively via questionnaire at child ages 5, 7, 9, and 11 years. Indicators of positive health domains including general health, physical health, and mental health were assessed and reported by mothers when their children were between the ages of 10-20 years and self-reported among a subset of children at 16-20 years. Children were grouped into "stressed" and "non-stressed" NQ groups based on the repeated prospective maternal report evaluating various aspects of their neighborhood. Overall, we found a general trend that those in the perceived "non-stressed" NQ groups had better Global Health compared to those in the "stressed" NQ group. In the subset of children who provided self-report, we observed significant associations between better overall NQ and NQ safety and better Global Health. We also observed a significant relationship between greater perceived neighborhood social cohesion and lower psychological stress. Our findings identify an important modifiable environmental factor in child and adolescent health that could serve as a focus for interventions to help break the cycle of children's environmental health disparities.

A grief group for today's teens: Using human-centered design to develop an evidence-based intervention for teens that have lost a parent

Trainee: Julia Chavez; Mentor: Dana Suskind; Institution: University of Chicago, Chicago, IL

Abstract: Parent loss during childhood is a profoundly stressful life event affecting one in 25 individuals in the United States. Early parent loss places children at risk for both short- and long-term negative health and life outcomes, including mental health issues (e.g., depression, anxiety, post-traumatic stress disorder) and lower academic success. Given the potential negative sequelae across the lifespan, timely intervention is critical. In this study, we used human-centered design (HCD) to develop an evidence-based intervention for teens who have lost a parent, using the Family Bereavement Program (FBP) as a model. A new peer-led delivery model was introduced to the curriculum, as well as the incorporation of technology and mindfulness strategies. We recruited researchers and members of the target population to provide feedback on the curriculum in focus groups. The results of focus group testing indicated that there are theory-practice gaps within post-bereavement interventions that can be identified and redressed through human-centered design framework. The focus group feedback provided preliminary support for the peer-led curriculum for parentally bereaved teens as well as suggestions for adaptation and modifications. Future work will be centered around further refining the model ensuring fidelity and scalability of the intervention.

Conclusion

The consequences of poverty on the health and well-being of children are clear in the dramatic disparities in health and access to quality healthcare. Income-related disparities are compounded and multiplied by the impact of racial disparities. The additional assault of COVID-19 on this vulnerable population of children, as well as long-term threat of climate change further exacerbates the health disparities. The human costs in loss of earning potential and the added economic costs to society in supporting such large populations of poor children in poor physical, social, and emotional health take its toll on the whole of society. It is incumbent upon all of us to recognize these disparities and inequities and develop strategies to reduce the disparities and promote health equity among all children. In this spirit, we offer a model for developing creative strategies while, at the same time, cultivating future leaders to make the critically necessary positive changes to our society.

As a core principle, *Break the Cycle* promotes awareness of the social, economic, and environmental determinants of health and encourages the development of creative and innovative strategies to reduce and eliminate health disparities in our society, for the good of all. As in previous *Break the Cycle* programs, current students benefited from the process of creatively developing a project, translating it into action, performing the research, presenting the results of their projects at a national conference, and writing manuscripts for publication in this journal. Each student project highlights ways to Break the Cycle of Children's Environmental Health Disparities through different components of the *Break the Cycle* diagram (see Figure 1):

- To reduce the likelihood of exposure to adverse environmental factors for vulnerable children,
- To improve their environmental circumstances by providing enhanced support, quality education and quality health care,
- To reduce added stressors, and,
- To promote resilience.

In this process, the students have gained valuable knowledge and skills towards becoming the next generation of leaders, and, building on their knowledge and experience, to further the goals of reducing children's environmental health disparities and promoting health equity for all children. This research and training model is a relatively inexpensive and cost-effective way of inspiring young bright students to focus their potential on changing the world for the better by developing research and communication skills and by embodying the principles of justice, equity, and collaboration. In the process, we all gain additional knowledge, understanding and perspective to become a more inclusive society and open to innovations and progress.

Acknowledgments

Thanks to the additional editors of some of the papers who have given of their time and expertise, much appreciated especially our trusted friend and star guest editor, editor David Ervin, as well as Erin Lebow-Skelly at the HERCULES Project at Emory University Rollins School of Public Health. This publication was supported by the cooperative agreement award number 5 NU61TS000237-05 from the Agency for Toxic Substances and Disease Registry (ATSDR). Its contents are the responsibility of the authors and do not necessarily represent the official views of the Agency for Toxic Substances and Disease Registry (ATSDR). The US Environmental Protection Agency (EPA) supports the PEHSU by providing partial funding to ATSDR under Inter-Agency Agreement number DW-75-95877701. Neither EPA nor ATSDR endorse the purchase of any commercial products or services mentioned in PEHSU publications.

References

[1] Etzel RA, Balk SJ, eds. Children's unique vulnerabilities to environmental hazards. In: Etzel RA, Balk SJ, eds. Pediatric environmental Health, 4th Edition: Itasca, IL: American Academy of Pediatrics, 2019:17-31.

[2] The Lancet Child Adolescent Health. Pollution: Think of the children. Lancet Child Adolesc Health 2017;1(4):249. https://doi.org/10.1016/S2352-4642(17)30133-5.

[3] Cooney CM. Stress-pollution interactions: an emerging issue in children's health research. Environ Health Perspect 2011;119(10):A431-5. doi:10.1289/ehp.119-a430CDC.

[4] Kim DY, Staley F, Curtis G, Buchanan S. Relation between housing age, housing value, and childhood blood lead levels in children in Jefferson County, KY. Am J Public Health 2002;92(5):769-72.

[5] Egan KB, Cornwell CR, Courtney JG, Ettinger AS. Blood lead levels in US children ages 1–11 years, 1976–2016. Environ Health Perspect 2021;129(3). https://doi.org/10.1289/EHP7932.

[6] Adamkiewicz G, Zota AR, Fabian MP, Chahine T, Julien R, Spengler JD, Levy JI. Moving environmental justice indoors: understanding structural influences on residential exposure patterns in low-income communities. Am J Public Health 2011;101(Suppl 1):S238–45.

[7] How do school funding formulas work? URL: https://apps.urban.org/features/funding-formulas/.

[8] Barshay, J. The Hechinger Report: A decade of research on the rich-poor divide in education. URL: https://hechingerreport.org/a-decade-of-research-on-the-rich-poor-divide-in-education/.

[9] Semuels A. Good school, rich school; bad school, poor school: The inequality at the heart of America's education system. The Atlantic 2016 Aug 25. URL: https://www.theatlantic.com/business/archive/2016/08/property-taxes-and-unequal-schools/497333/.

[10] Solomon GM, Morello-Frosch R, Zeise L, Faust JB. Cumulative environmental impacts: Science and policy to protect communities. Annu Rev Public Health 2016;37:83–96.

[11] Faust JB. Perspectives on cumulative risks and impacts. Int J Toxicol 2010;29(1):58-64.

[12] Pacheco CM, Ciaccio CE, Nazir M, Daley CM, DiDonna A,4 Won S. Choi, Barnes CS, P Rosenwasser LJ. Homes of low-income minority families with asthmatic children have increased condition issues. Allergy Asthma Proc 2014;35(6):467–74.

[13] Healthy People 2020. URL: https://www.healthypeople.gov/2020/topics-objectives/topic/social-determinants-health/interventions-resources/quality-of-housing.

[14] National Environmental Justice Advisory Council. Cumulative Risks/Impacts Work Group. Ensuring risk reduction in communities with multiple stressors: Environmental justice and cumulative risks/impacts, 2004. URL: https://www.epa.gov/sites/production/files/2015-04/documents/ensuringriskreducationnejac.pdf.

[15] Pair QC, Environmental justice and the future of America. Int Public Health J 2021;13(4):377-88.
[16] Hodgkinson S, Godoy L, Beers LS. Improving mental health access for low-income children and families in the primary care setting. Pediatrics 2017;139(1):e20151175.
[17] Shonkoff JP, Garner AS, Committee on Psychosocial Aspects of Child and Family Health, Committee on Early Childhood, Adoption, and Dependent Care, Section on Developmental and Behavioral Pediatrics. The lifelong effects of early childhood adversity and toxic stress. Pediatrics 2012;129(1):e232-46.
[18] Hood E. Dwelling disparities: How poor housing leads to poor health. Environ Health Perspect 2005;113(5):A310–17.
[19] Friedman J, Karandinos G, Hart LK, Castrillo FM, Graetz N. Structural vulnerability to narcotics-driven firearm violence: An ethnographic and epidemiological study of Philadelphia's Puerto Rican inner-city. PLoS One 2019;14(11):e0225376.
[20] Rubin IL, Geller RJ, Martinuzzi K, Howett M, Gitterman BA, Wells LM, et al. Children's environmental health disparities: The costs and benefits of breaking the cycle. Int J Child Health Hum Dev 2016;9(4):419-30.
[21] The Sentencing Project. Criminal Justice facts. URL: https://www.sentencingproject.org/criminal-justice-facts/.
[22] Sickmund M, Sladky TJ, Puzzanchera C, Kang W. Easy access to the Census of Juveniles in Residential Placement, 2021. URL: https://www.ojjdp.gov/ojstatbb/ezacjrp/.
[23] Rubin IL. Resilience: A commentary on breaking the cycle. Int Public Health J 2018;10(3):247-64.
[24] Wodtke GT, Elwert F, Harding DJ. Poor families, poor neighborhoods: How family poverty intensifies the impact of concentrated disadvantage on high school graduation. Ann Arbor, MI: University Michigan, Population Studies Center Research Report 12-776, 2012.
[25] Mood C, Jonsson JO. The social consequences of poverty: An empirical test on longitudinal data. Soc Indic Res 2016;127:633–52.
[26] Rubin IL, Geller RJ, Martinuzzi K, Howett M, Gitterman BA, Wells L, et al. Break the cycle of children's environmental health disparities. An ecological framework. Int Public Health J 2017;9(2):115-249.
[27] Pascoe JM, Wood DL, Duffee JH. AAP Committee on Psychosocial Aspects of Child and Family Health, Council on Community Pediatrics. Mediators and Adverse Effects of Child Poverty in the United States. Pediatrics 2016;137(4):e20160340.
[28] Children's Defense Fund. State of American Children. URL: https://www.childrensdefense.org/wp-content/uploads/2020/02/The-State-Of-Americas-Children-2020.pdf.
[29] CDC. Infant mortality. URL: https://www.cdc.gov/reproductivehealth/maternalinfanthealth/infantmortality.htm.
[30] Lee C. Confronting disproportionate impacts and systemic racism in environmental policy. Environ Law Reporter 2021 March 10.
[31] Johnson TJ. Intersection of bias, structural racism, and social determinants with health care inequities. Pediatrics 2020;146(2):e2020003657.

[32] CDC. Health equity. Racism and health. UR: https://www.cdc.gov/healthequity/racism-disparities/index.html.
[33] Trent M, Dooley DG, Dougé J. The impact of racism on child and adolescent health. Pediatrics 2019;144(2):e20191765.
[34] Garg S, Kim L, Whitaker M. Hospitalization rates and characteristics of patients hospitalized with laboratory-confirmed Coronavirus disease 2019 — COVID-NET, 14 States, March 1–30, 2020. MMWR 2020;69:458–64.
[35] Yancy CW. COVID-19 and African Americans. JAMA 2020 Apr 15. doi:10.1001/jama.2020.6548.
[36] CDC. Introduction to COVID-19 racial and ethnic health disparities. URL: https://www.cdc.gov/coronavirus/2019-ncov/community/health-equity/racial-ethnic-disparities/index.html.
[37] Chowkwanyun M, Reed AL. Racial health disparities and Covid-19: Caution and context. N Engl J Med 2020;383:201-3.
[38] Framing a discourse on health disparities and social inequities. Public Adm Rev 2020;80(5):839–44.
[39] Alcendor J. Racial disparities-associated COVID-19 mortality among minority populations in the US. J Clin Med 2020;9(8):2442.
[40] Mude W, Oguoma VM, Nyanhanda T, Mwanri L, Njue C. Racial disparities in COVID-19 pandemic cases, hospitalisations, and deaths: A systematic review and meta-analysis. J Glob Health. 2021;11:05015.
[41] American Academy of Pediatrics. Children and COVID-19: State-level data report. URL: https://www.aap.org/en/pages/2019-novel-coronavirus-covid-19-infections/children-and-covid-19-state-level-data-report/.
[42] CDC. Multisystem inflammatory syndrome in children (MIS-C): Information for healthcare providers about talking with families and caregivers. URL: https://www.cdc.gov/mis/mis-c/hcp/provider-families.html#:~:text=Studies%20have%20reported%20that%20MIS,SARS%2DCoV%2D2%20infection.
[43] Stierman B, Abrams JY, Godfred-Cato SE, Oster ME, Meng L, Yip L, et al. Racial and ethnic disparities in multisystem inflammatory syndrome in children in the United States, March 2020 to February 2021. Pediatr Infect Dis J 2021;40(11):e400-6.
[44] UNICEF. COVID-19 and children. URL: https://data.unicef.org/covid-19-and-children/.
[45] NIH. More than 140,000 US children lost a primary or secondary caregiver due to the COVID-19 pandemic. URL: https://www.nih.gov/news-events/news-releases/more-140000-us-children-lost-primary-or-secondary-caregiver-due-covid-19-pandemic.
[46] Hillis SD, Blenkinsop A, Villaveces A, Annor FB, Liburd L, Massetti GM, et al. COVID-19-associated orphanhood and caregiver death in the United States. Pediatrics 2021. doi: 10.1542/peds.2021-053760.
[47] NOAA. Climate change: Global temperature URL: https://www.climate.gov/news-features/understanding-climate/climate-change-global-temperature#:~:text=Earth's%20temperature%20has%20risen%20by,land%20areas%20were%20record%20warm.

[48] Smith CJ. Pediatric thermoregulation: Considerations in the face of global climate change. Nutrients 2019;11(9):2010.

[49] Bergeron MF, Devore C, Rice SG. Policy statement--climatic heat stress and exercising children and adolescents. Pediatrics 2011;128(3):e741-7.

[50] EPA. Learn about heat islands. URL: https://www.epa.gov/heatislands/learn-about-heat-islands#:~:text=A%20review%20of%20research%20studies,2%E2%80%935%C2%B0F%20higher.

[51] Gronlund CJ. Racial and socioeconomic disparities in heat-related health effects and their mechanisms: a review. Curr Epidemiol Rep 2014;1(3):165–73.

[52] NOAA. National Centers for Environmental Information. US. 2021 billion-dollar weather and climate disasters. URL: https://www.ncdc.noaa.gov/billions/.

[53] Lai BS, La Greca A. Understanding the impacts of natural disasters on children. Society for Research in Child Development. Child Evidence Brief No 8, 2020. URL: https://www.srcd.org/research/understanding-impacts-natural-disasters-children.

[54] Rubin IL, Falk H, Mutic A. Natural disasters and vulnerable populations: a commentary. Int J Child Health Hum Dev 2019;12(4):303-18.

[55] Makwana N. Disaster and its impact on mental health: a narrative review. J Fam Med Prim Care 2019;8(10):3090-5.

[56] Rubin IL, Oves D, Nodvin J, Geller RJ, Howett M, Martinuzzi K, et al. The learning experience of 'Break the Cycle' program: Survey of past students. In: Rubin IL, Merrick J, eds. Environmental health disparities. New York: Nova Science, 2016:171-85.

Section one: BTC in time of COVID-19

Chapter 2

An examination of the prevalence of COVID-19 in the Texas Juvenile Justice System

Rachel J Slover[1,*] and Rebecca Fry[2], PhD

[1]University of North Carolina at Chapel Hill, Chapel Hill, North Carolina, United States of America

[2]Department of Environmental Sciences and Engineering, Gilling School of Global Public Health, University of North Carolina at Chapel Hill, Chapel Hill, North Carolina, United States of America

Abstract

COVID-19 has posed a nationwide public health emergency, and one of the most at-risk yet concurrently overlooked populations in the United States has been youth in the juvenile justice system. In order to understand how to break the cycle of environmental health disparities faced by incarcerated youth, an examination was performed of the prevalence of COVID-19 in the juvenile justice system through a Texas case study – chosen due to the state's large incarcerated youth population, vulnerability to COVID-19, and transparency in data reporting. Data on demographics and COVID-19 case counts were gathered on Texas Juvenile Justice Department (TJJD) facilities to understand who comprises the at-risk population and the extent of that risk. The potential for community influence on facility vulnerability was examined through data from the NIEHS Pandemic Vulnerability Index (PVI) and data from the TJJD on staff COVID-19 case counts. Analysis found racial disparities between placement in high versus lower-security TJJD facilities and between the state and TJJD population compositions. Findings further demonstrated baseline TJJD county vulnerability, high COVID-19 case counts for incarcerated youth, likely disease vectors

* *Correspondence*: Rachel J Slover, University of North Carolina at Chapel Hill, Chapel Hill, North Carolina, United States. Email: rachel.j.slover@gmail.com.

In: Environmental Health

Editors: I Leslie Rubin and Joav Merrick

ISBN: 979-8-88697-292-4

from the staff to the youth, and disparities in case counts between facilities. Further research should be conducted to assess the sources of the disparities and how to best inform methods to break the cycle of health disparities and strive for equitable youth justice.

Introduction

The COVID-19 pandemic created a significant risk to environmental public health in the United States, with over 34 million reported cases and over 608,800 deaths by July 2021 (1). Research has indicated that different populations are disproportionately affected by and at risk for COVID-19, with disparities connected to factors such as income, race, geographic location, population density, and pre-existing medical conditions (2, 3).

Congregate settings are especially at risk for increased disease spread, which leaves incarcerated youth at a higher risk than their nonincarcerated counterparts. In regard to their heightened vulnerability, Dr Craig W. Haney, an expert on the psychological effects of incarceration at UC Santa Cruz, wrote in a March 2020 court statement that, when thinking of incarcerated people, including incarcerated youth, "it is thus hard to imagine a more vulnerable population … in the face of this pandemic," (4). While COVID-19 is not typically as severe for children as for adults, research is still unclear as to the long-term health outcomes of past pediatric COVID-19 infections, so even asymptomatic or mild cases in children may bring negative consequences in adult life.

This risk of COVID-19 only adds to the significant disparities already faced by incarcerated youth. According to the American Academy of Family Physicians, incarcerated youth have higher morbidity and mortality rates than the general adolescent population, and two-thirds of incarcerated boys and more than four-fifths of incarcerated girls meet the criteria for at least one mental health disorder (5). As such, incarcerated youth have much higher baseline rates of underlying health conditions that put them at greater risk for COVID-19. These pre-existing factors may also put them at greater risk of developing mental health disorders post-COVID-19 infection (6). These risks disproportionately faced by incarcerated youth are represented in Figure 1. These children face risks such as but not limited to: increased isolation, increased exposure to disease outbreaks, increased rates of mental health conditions, disruption to education, limited healthcare, poverty, increased likelihood of adult incarceration, and family disruption – factors that all compound and keep them trapped in a cycle of health disparities. Though overall juvenile justice populations have been steadily declining in recent years, population density is still too high to effectively protect youth from disease contraction and spread (7).

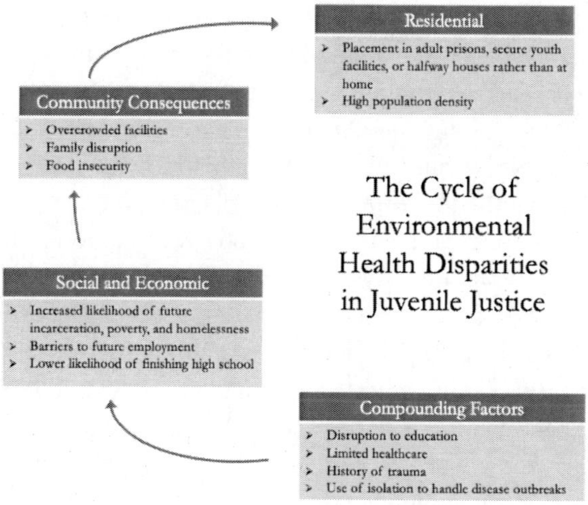

Figure 1. The cycle of environmental health disparities in juvenile justice. The cycle of environmental health disparities faced by youth in the juvenile justice system, separated by category of disparity and potential examples. The order of effect can differ, but the cyclical nature of the consequences is enduring.

While states have taken measures to mitigate the impact of COVID-19, these policies often create new issues. In an attempt to prevent the spread of COVID-19, many juvenile facilities have undertaken severe isolation measures akin to solitary confinement – usually illegal and considered inhumane in juvenile justice. Children can be locked in isolation cells for twenty-three hours each day, only able to interact with corrections officers, shouting to their friends under their cell doors (8). Incarcerated youth are left feeling scared and alone, especially as they are often deprived of information and isolated from their loved ones due to cancellation of visitation, activities, and in-person education (9). The American Academy of Pediatrics has urged that continuing these inhumane practices must be considered a dire health emergency (10).

The Society for Adolescent Health and Medicine followed suit by urging juvenile justice departments to "Release youth who can be safely cared for in their home communities" (10). While many states attempted this tactic, it was not done equitably. According to a monthly survey of juvenile justice agencies in more than 30 states conducted by the Annie E Casey Foundation, by May 2020, White youths were released at a 17% higher rate than Black youths (11). Further, while the number of White youths has remained at a historic low in the months since the initial survey, the number of Black and Latino youths has risen, and Black and Latino youths are being detained longer than they were pre-pandemic (11). Experts suggest that this could be attributed to bias in sentencing, young people of color having higher rates of detention for serious offenses, or their communities lacking alternatives to incarceration (11). This disparity in racial and ethnic release rates from early in the pandemic suggests need for further investigation into rates of release and detention across racial and ethnic groups at the end of the pandemic's surge/post-vaccination in late 2020 and early 2021.

Texas was selected for case study due to the large juvenile justice population, better data availability, and better data reliability. Texas has a commitment rate of 67 per 100,000 juveniles ages 10 and up, compared to the US average of 66, and a detention rate of 59 per 100,000 juveniles ages 10 and up, compared to the U.S. average of 45, and therefore represents a larger portion of the nation's at-risk incarcerated youth (12). Further, Texas is one of the systems with the most available data, as they publicly post a timeline of COVID-19 diagnoses and readily shared further data when requested, while many other state juvenile justice departments have released little to no data about their COVID-19 safety measures, case counts, or testing. Finally, TJJD COVID-19 data was possibly more reliable than that of many other states because Texas is one of the few states whose juvenile justice department announced plans to perform comprehensive testing of all incarcerated youth within state-run facilities.

In their COVID-19 mitigation policies, TJJD reported implemen-tation of protective policies against COVID-19, including, but not limited to: everyone who enters the facility receives a health screening and a temperature check; new youth are masked until they can be assessed; symptomatic youth are moved to medical quarantine; sanitation measures were increased through hand washing, staff masking, and frequent cleaning; and changes were made to social interaction, requiring youth to remain in small groups with no social crossover, cancelling visitation, and holding education in dorms in smaller groups rather than in the school (13).

This research investigated the demographics of the TJJD population, the vulnerability of the geographic locations where these facilities are located, rates of COVID-19 infection at different TJJD facilities, and how staff case counts compared to youth case counts, in order to better inform potential methods to break the cycle of health disparities faced by incarcerated youth.

Our study

A preliminary data search was performed to investigate which state juvenile justice systems had sections of their websites related to COVID-19. Due to time constraints, only five states (California, Florida, Georgia, South Carolina, and Texas) were contacted via email to request additional data. Only representatives from Texas responded and provided sufficient data, so the investigation moved forward with Texas.

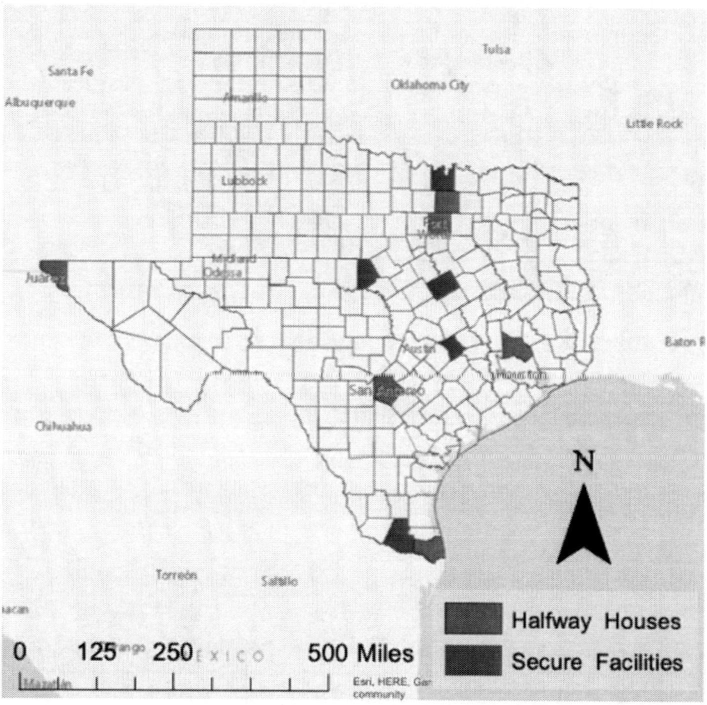

Figure 2. Map of TJJD facility counties.
The counties where each facility is located are mapped above, with halfway house counties in blue and secure facility counties in purple. County populations range from approximately 17,000 to over 2 million, representing varied population size and density across community locations.

The TJJD provided data on their eleven state-run facilities: five secure facilities and six halfway houses (see Figure 2). Though the TJJD population also includes youth on parole and youth in contract facilities (privately run facilities, which are common nationwide), COVID-19 data was not accessible for these populations, so data collection was limited to secure facilities and halfway houses.

Census data from 2019 was gathered for each of the eleven counties where the TJJD facilities are located, which provided reasonable estimates for 2020/2021 data (14). This included: county population, percent African American/Black alone, percent Hispanic/Latino, percent White alone (not Hispanic/Latino), and percent other.

Table 1. Gender and age across the TJJD

	All State-Operated Residential & Halfway Houses (n = 659)	**Evins Regional Juvenile Center (n = 45)**	**Gainesville State School (n = 116)**	**Giddings State School (n = 136)**	**McLennan County State Juvenile Correctional Facility (n = 194)**	**Ron Jackson State Juvenile Correctional Facility (n = 121)**	**Halfway Houses (n = 47)**
Male (%)	91.70%	91.50%	100.00%	100.00%	100.00%	56.19%	93.62%
Female (%)	8.30%	8.50%	0.00%	0.00%	0.00%	43.80%	6.38%
Age (Mean)	16.65	16.58	16.81	16.94	16.56	16.33	16.77

Table 2. Race and ethnicity in TJJD versus Texas state total

	Black		**Hispanic**		**White**		**Other**	
	All Facilities	**State Total**	**All Facilities**	**State Total**	**All Facilities**	**State Total**	**All Facilities**	**State Total**
All Secure Facilities (n = 612)	41.01%	12.90%	43.80%	39.70%	18.18%	41.20%	1.65%	8.40%
Halfway Houses (n = 47)	17.02%		40.43%		42.55%		0.00%	
All State-Operated Residential & Halfway Houses (n = 659)	39.30%		41.27%		18.51%		0.91%	

The TJJD provided data via email, on age, race/ethnicity, and gender for 1/31/2021, and on population of each facility for four dates: 6/30/2020,

8/31/2020, 12/31/2020, and 1/31/2021. Demographic data was analyzed in Excel to examine trends across facilities and to compare TJJD demographics to the state of Texas overall (see Tables 1-2), and population data was examined and recorded (see Table 3).

Table 3. TJJD population

		Population			
		June 30th, 2020	**August 31st, 2020**	**December 31st, 2020**	**January 31st, 2021**
State-Operated Secure Facilities	Evins Regional Juvenile Center	113	102	41	45
	Gainesville State School	111	93	114	116
	Giddings State School	191	142	140	136
	McLennan County State Juvenile Correctional Facility	202	174	161	194
	Ron Jackson State Juvenile Correctional Complex	81	97	119	121
	Subtotal Type	698	608	575	612
Halfway Houses	Ayres House	10	10	12	6
	Karyn's House	5	4	3	3
	McFadden Ranch	23	18	17	18
	Schaeffer House	10	6	6	2
	Tamayo House	13	8	12	11
	Willoughby House	9	9	6	7
	Subtotal Type	70	55	56	47
Total State-Operated Residential		768	663	631	659

County data was drawn from the NIEHS COVID-19 Pandemic Vulnerability Index (PVI) (15). The PVI provides a normalized "PVI" score that acts as a representation of the vulnerability of each county in the country and ranks all counties from most to least vulnerable, while providing a "ToxPi" chart, or visualization of vulnerability, for each county. The PVI assessed four different categories in determining overall vulnerability: infection rates, intervention rates, population concentration and density, and health and environmental variables. Toxicological Priority Index (ToxPi) charts, PVI scores, and Texas-wide and national vulnerability rankings were gathered for each facility county as well as for Newton county, a county with similar population size but a lower PVI score, as comparison (see Figure 3). This served to represent the vulnerability of each county.

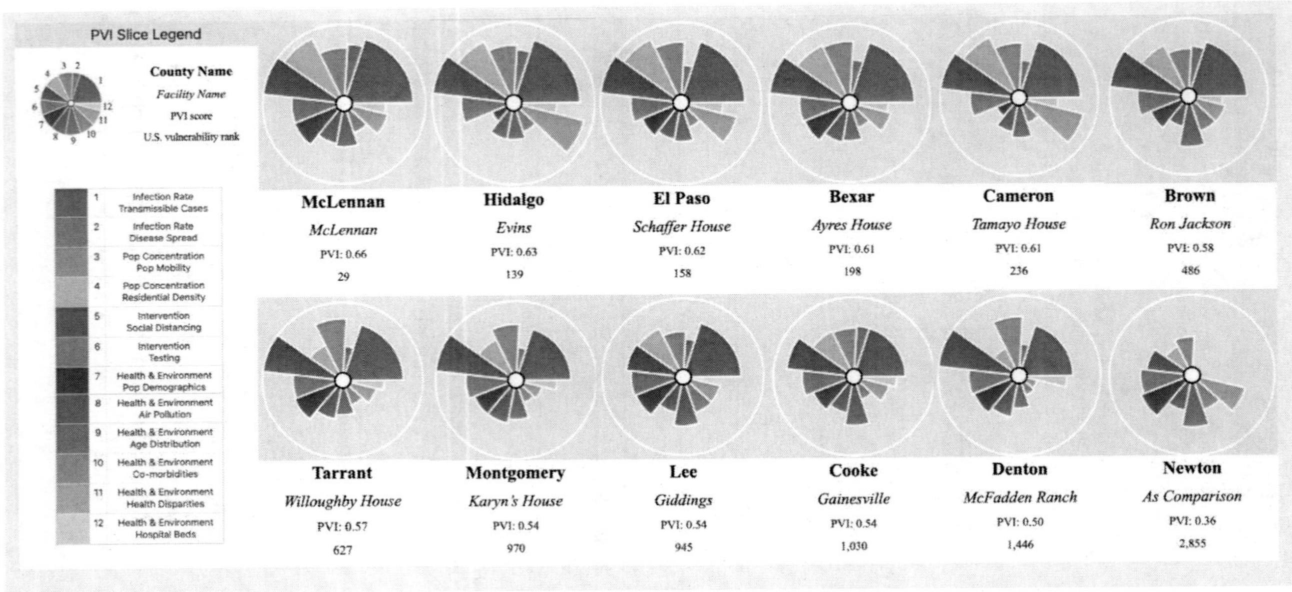

Figure 3. NIEHS Pandemic Vulnerability Index (PIV) ToxPi charts.
Each of the 11 TJJD counties alongside the example of a less-vulnerable county, Newton, Texas, organized from most to least vulnerable (top to bottom, left to right). The PVI is a normalized score representing vulnerability, with 0 being the least and 1 being the most vulnerable. Each slice represents a different vulnerability metric from the legend to the right; the reds (1, 2) represent disease transmission, the greens (3, 4) population density, the blues (5, 6) interventions, and the purples (7-12) environmental and health vulnerabilities. The distance from the center of each slice is proportional to the value of that metric while the width of each slice is proportional to the weight of that metric in the overall PVI calculation.

Table 4. Youth COVID-19 case counts

		Youth Cumulative COVID-19 Cases				Youth New COVID-19 Cases				Youth Percent of Population with a New COVID-19 Case (%)			
		6/30 2020	**8/31 2020**	**8/31 2020**	**1/31 2021**	**6/30 2020**	**8/31 2020**	**8/31 2020**	**1/31 2021**	**6/30 2020**	**8/31 2020**	**8/31 2020**	**1/31 2021**
State-Operated Secure Facilities	Evins Regional Juvenile Center	3	31	45	45	3	28	14	0	2.65%	27.45%	34.15%	0%
	Gainesville State School	8	13	13	13	8	5	0	0	7.21%	5.38%	0%	0%
	Giddings State School	11	84	99	107	11	73	15	8	5.76%	51.41%	10.71%	5.88%
	McLennan County State Juvenile Correctional Facility	0	42	98	102	0	42	56	4	0%	24.14%	34.78%	2.06%
	Ron Jackson State Juvenile Correctional Complex	0	26	30	30	0	26	4	0	0%	26.80%	3.36%	0%
	Subtotal Type	22	196	285	297	22	174	89	12	3.15%	28.62%	15.48%	1.96%
Halfway Houses	Subtotal Type	4	21	22	22	4	17	1	0	5.71%	30.91%	1.79%	0%

Table 5. Staff COVID-19 case counts

		Staff Cumulative COVID-19 Cases				Staff New COVID-19 Cases			
		6/30 2020	**8/31 2020**	**8/31 2020**	**1/31 2021**	**6/30 2020**	**8/31 2020**	**8/31 2020**	**1/31 2021**
State-Operated Secure Facilities	Evins Regional Juvenile Center	16	57	79	89	16	41	22	10
	Gainesville State School	4	11	26	38	4	7	15	12
	Giddings State School	7	39	67	87	7	32	28	20
	McLennan County State Juvenile Correctional Facility	0	23	79	103	0	23	56	24
	Ron Jackson State Juvenile Correctional Complex	6	41	71	81	6	35	30	10
	Subtotal Type	33	171	322	398	33	138	151	76
Halfway Houses	Subtotal Type	29	43	44	44	29	14	1	0

Cumulative and new (non-cumulative) COVID-19 case counts for youth and staff for each of the four dates were determined based on the TJJD's public timeline of new COVID-19 cases (13). This data was recorded (see Tables 4 and 5), analyzed, and used to calculate percent of youth population with a positive test result in each timeframe. COVID-19 case counts were then plotted across facilities for both youth and staff to identify trends (see Figures 4-6). New youth and staff case counts were used to assess correlation and plot timelines between youth and staff case counts at each facility (see Figure 7).

All TJJD press releases from March 2020 through March 2021 were reviewed and significant updates were recorded to construct timelines of potentially significant events, number of cumulative youth tests performed, and case counts throughout the pandemic. Days with high case counts (>10) were marked. Dates of significant Texas state COVID-19 policies were also recorded from the website of the Office of the Texas Governor press releases (16). Identified dates were examined alongside timelines of case peaks to assess possible relationships.

Our findings

Examination of the gender and age distribution of the TJJD is provided in Table 1 and shows that the TJJD population in January 2021 was overwhelmingly male at 91.5% and only 8.5% female. The mean age was consistent across all facilities at approximately 16.5-17 years old.

Table 2 displays the findings of the analysis of the racial and ethnic composition of the TJJD compared to the state total. Primary analysis returned evidence of disparity in placement in high versus lower security facilities. Black youth comprised 41.0% of secure facility populations, yet comprised only 17.0% of halfway house populations. White youth were found to have nearly the opposite placement, making up 18.2% of secure facility populations and 42.6% of halfway house populations. Additionally, overall disparities were found between the TJJD population and the state population; though Black youth accounted for only 12.9% of the state population, they comprised 39.3% of the TJJD population, whereas White youth accounted for 41.2% of the state population yet only comprised 18.5% of the TJJD population. Findings for Hispanic youth were consistent across facility types and consistent in the comparison of state versus TJJD populations, all ranging from 40.4% to 43.8%.

NIEHS PVI

Analysis of the NIEHS COVID-19 PVI from July 13, 2020, highlighted the heightened level of vulnerability that each of these counties faced overall, which potentially translates to higher vulnerability for youth, as staff likely live in the surrounding counties. Figure 3 shows each of the eleven TJJD counties alongside the example of a less-vulnerable county, Newton, Texas, ranked from most to least vulnerable based on PVI score. The PVI score is a normalized value representing vulnerability, with 0 being the least and 1 being the most vulnerable. All of the PVI scores of the TJJD counties are higher than average, ranging from 0.50 to 0.63. Additionally, many of the TJJD counties ranked high in nationwide vulnerability (ranging from 139th to 1,446th out of 3,142 total counties analyzed nationwide) and in Texas-wide vulnerability (ranging from 5th to 169th out of 259 total counties in Texas). In comparison, Newton has a PVI score of 0.36 and a nationwide ranking of 2,855. The most vulnerable county was McLennan, where McLennan County State Juvenile Correctional Facility is located, with a PVI score of 0.66 and a ranking of 29.

Population

TJJD population data is compiled in Table 3. The two most populated facilities in June 2020 were McLennan County State Juvenile Correctional Facility (McLennan) and Giddings State School (Giddings) with populations of 202 and 191 respectively, followed by Evins Regional Juvenile Center (Evins) with 113, Gainesville State School (Gainesville) with 111, and Ron Jackson State Juvenile Correctional Complex (Ron Jackson) with 81. Halfway house populations ranged from 2 to 25, with a total June 2020 population of 70, and ending with a total January 2021 population of 47 – a 32.9% decrease. McLennan and Gainesville maintained fairly consistent populations throughout the examined period; McLennan's population increased by only 3.9% to 194, and Gainesville's population increased by only 4.5% to 116. Evins decreased their population by 60.2%, going from 113 in June 2020 to 45 in January 2021. Giddings decreased their population by 28.8%, with their January 2021 population down from 191 to 136. Ron Jackson increased their population by 49.4%, going from 81 in June 2020 to 121 in January 2021.

Youth and staff case counts

Youth case counts corresponding to these population changes are displayed in Table 4. Across the entire TJJD, 297 youth cases were logged by January 1, 2021. The most significant increase in this period occurred between June 30, 2020, and August 31, 2020, with a 691% increase in new (non-cumulative) cases from 22 to 174. This was the period of the greatest number of new cases. The greatest number of youth cases were found at Giddings and McLennan, with 107 and 102 cumulative cases respectively, while the other facilities all maintained under 50 cases total (see Figure 4). These case counts were over 50% higher than other facilities.

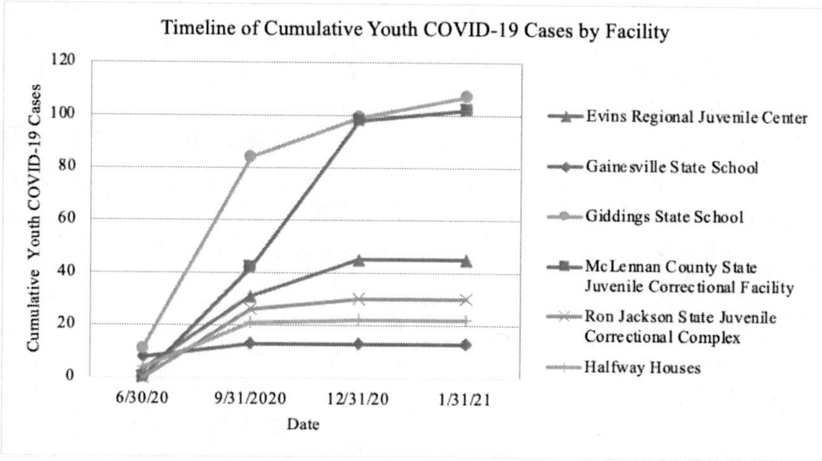

Figure 4. Cumulative youth COVID-19 cases from June 2020 to January 2021 by facility.

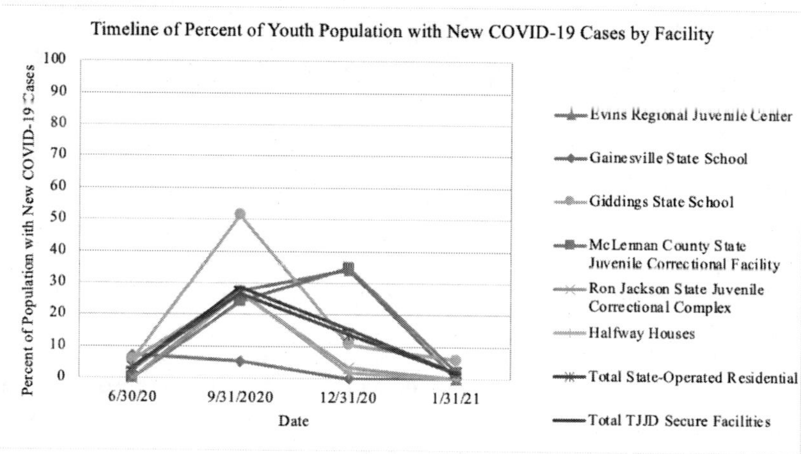

Figure 5. Percent of the youth population with new COVID-19 cases from June 2020 to January 2021 by facility.

When adjusted for differences in population by logging new cases as percent of population (see Figure 5), Giddings still had a greater percent of youth contracting COVID-19, with 51.4% of the population having contracted COVID-19 between June and August 2020. Once adjusted for population, McLennan has a similar infection percentage to Ron Jackson, Evins, and all Halfway Houses, with each having 24-29% of their population contracting

COVID-19 between June and August 2020. While Ron Jackson and McLennan follow nearly identical trajectories into December and January, Ron Jackson's infection rate decreases significantly in December 2020 from 26.8% to 3.4%. Gainesville was able to maintain low youth COVID-19 case counts, from 7.2% in June 2020 to 5.4% in August 2020, reaching and maintaining zero by December 31, 2020. Though Ron Jackson and Halfway Houses were also near zero by December 2020, Gainesville was the only facility with no reported spike in cases in August 2020.

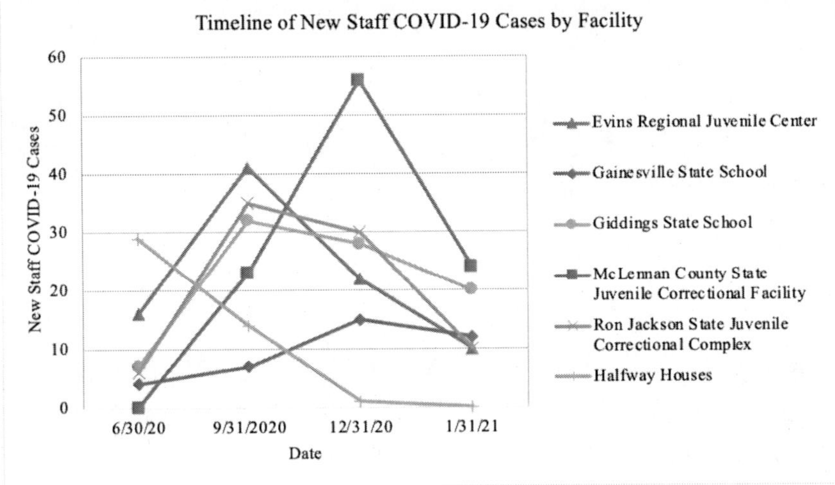

Figure 6. New staff COVID-19 cases from June 2020 to January 2021 by facility.

Data on cumulative and new staff cases is compiled in Table 5. A similar pattern to the youth outcome is seen with new staff cases, with 398 total identified cases by January 31, 2021 and a 318% increase between June 30, 2020 and August 31, 2020 from 33 to 138. Unlike youth cases, this was only the second highest period of new cases, as most new staff cases occurred between August 31 and December 31, 2020, with 151. The most staff cases were found at McLennan, with 103 by January 2021, followed by Evins, Giddings, and Ron Jackson all in the mid-eighties, with the lowest at Gainesville, with only 38 cumulative cases. As with youth, the most significant contraction period for staff was between June and August 2020, increasing by 318% from 33 new cases to 138 new cases for the TJJD secure facilities as a whole. However, whereas new youth cases decreased between August and December 2020 from 174 to 89, new staff cases continued to increase, from 138 to 151. Visualization of these staff trends is provided in Figure 6.

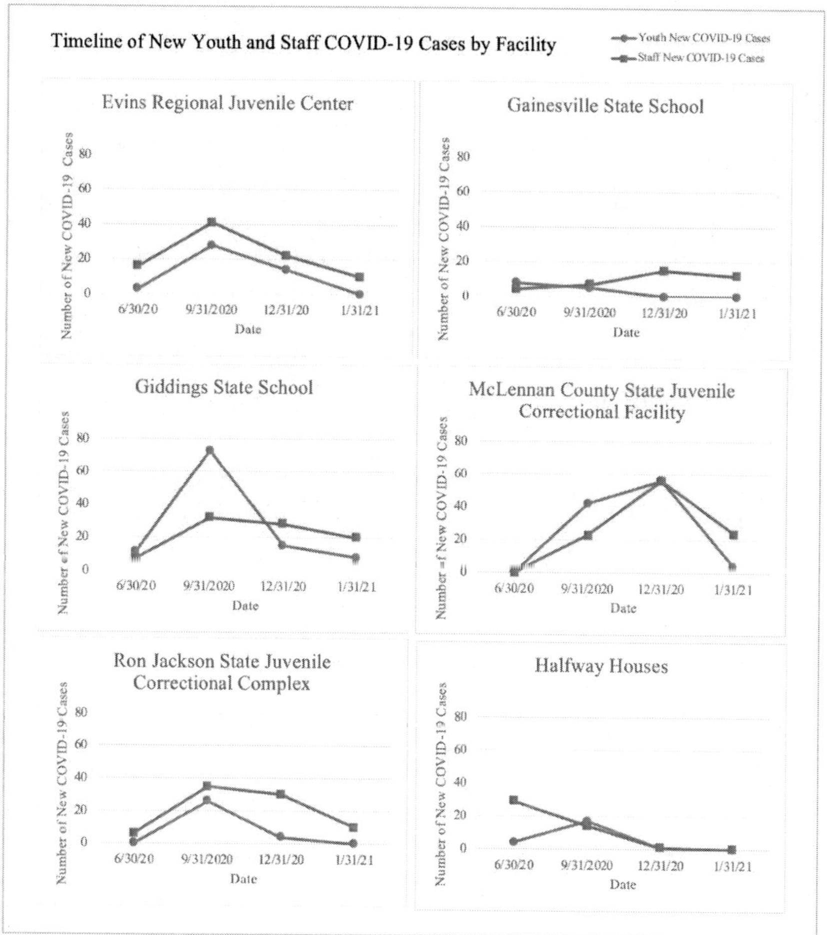

Figure 7. Relationship between youth and staff new cases by facility.

Plotting of youth and staff new case counts at each facility demonstrated possible correlation (see Figure 7). The most useful plot elements are the trajectories rather than the magnitudes, as no population data for number of staff was provided. For example, Giddings, may appear to have experienced a much greater spike in August for youth than staff, yet as staff population is likely inherently lower than youth population, this is less useful information that the fact that plots such as McLennan, Evins, and Ron Jackson, which show cases following roughly the same trajectory of maximums and minimums.

Timeline of important dates in TJJD and the surrounding communities

July 1, 2020: TJJD announces the beginning of campus-wide testing for all youth, tests are conducted through July 17th. *Coincides with August 31st.*

July 2, 2020: Texas Governor orders mask mandate in public spaces and bans gatherings over 10 people (with several exceptions). *Coincides with August 31st- December 30th.*

July 13, 2020: 29 youth cases are found at McLennan before campus-wide testing occurs. *Coincides with August 31st.*

September 17, 2020: Public schools and drive-ins can operate at full capacity; restaurants, retail, offices, manufacturers, museums, libraries, and gyms can operate at 75% capacity unless located in an area with high hospitalization rates. *Coincides with August 31st- December 30th.*

December 19, 2020: 16 youth cases are found at McLennan before campus-wide testing occurs. *Coincides with January 31st.*

January 11, 2021: TJJD announces the beginning of campus-wide testing for all youth as a post-holiday precaution, testing concludes on January 13th. *Coincides with January 31st.*

Discussion

Findings point to many vulnerabilities present in the cycle of environmental health disparities in juvenile justice (see Figure 1). From the NIEHS PVI analysis results, we can see that TJJD facilities were often located in already-vulnerable counties for disease spread, which could translate to heightened "Residential" vulnerability for the incarcerated youth. However, results indicate that while county vulnerability can have an effect, there are many other factors at work, for despite both Giddings' and Gainesville's county PVI scores being the same, they represented both extremes of the case count spectrum.

Analysis of staff and youth case counts, and findings of possible correlation support the potential for disease vectors both from the youth to the staff and from the staff to the youth via the surrounding community, increasing vulnerability across many categories (e.g., Residential, Environmental, Health Outcomes).

High youth infection percentages overall provide support for previous hypotheses that juvenile facilities have a high likelihood of disease spread that leaves these youth uniquely vulnerable to negative health outcomes.

While it is unclear from this investigation if these trends scale across the country or the degree of effect one factor has on the other, the potential influence should be given further attention and should factor into incarcerated youth disease mitigation planning.

Policy

Disparities in youth case counts of COVID-19 infections across facilities demonstrate a need for transparency in individual facility disease outbreak policies to assess why facilities like Gainesville were able to keep cases so low while others like Giddings experienced such surges. This further suggests the need for stronger standardized protection plans in juvenile justice departments to inform equitable protection. If a similar situation were to arise in the future, states must all adopt a policy of frequent comprehensive testing to ensure cases are rapidly identified. States should also publicize their population, demographic, and de-identified disease case count data in order to better enable accurate research into the prevalence of disease outbreaks.

Additionally, since burgeoning research points to previously unforeseen long term negative health outcomes for those who have recovered from COVID-19, future research should investigate the health outcomes for previously-incarcerated youth post-COVID-19 infection when compared with nonincarcerated youth.

The impact of the COVID-19 pandemic on incarcerated youth calls for reevaluation of the best way to provide true rehabilitation and support to incarcerated youth at such a pivotal point in their development. In order to draw clear conclusions, better data collection and publicization must become ubiquitous to facilitate more frequent and thorough research.

Limitations

It must be noted that limited data availability hinders the strength of possible conclusions from these findings. Data on population was only received for four dates, which likely oversimplifies the rapid turnover at many youth facilities. Data also did not specify which changes in youth population were due to newly sentenced youth versus youth transferred between facilities, which adds uncertainty in the risk of disease exposure between facilities. Population of staff at each facility was also unknown, and as such, the percent of staff infected was uncertain, as was the amount of contact that infected staff had with youth. This further underscores the need for better data reporting.

Further, while the PVI provides a useful baseline representation of county vulnerability and therefore potential risk of staff infection, vulnerability is influenced by more metrics than are analyzed here. For example, the PVI did not consider racial or ethnic demographics, income, access to health care, education level, etc. – all of which could provide more detailed information on vulnerability influencers and provide a more complete understanding of the variables in each county. These additional significant vulnerabilities and racial disparities are endemic to the juvenile justice system, not only in Texas, but nationwide, and result in youth of color being put at disproportionate risk which was not reflected in the data.

Additionally, the level of interaction that facility staff have with the surrounding county is unknown and could be variable between different counties, as it is unknown how many staff live in the surrounding counties. This affects the strength of the assumption that county vulnerability is related to staff and therefore youth vulnerability.

Though COVID-19 policies were reported for the TJJD as a whole, no direct communication was possible with any youth in the facilities nor any staff, so the degree to which these policies were consistently followed is uncertain, and any updates made to policies that were not listed on the TJJD website are unknown.

Additionally, though the insights gained from this investigation can prove useful for creating a framework for future research, different state juvenile justice departments followed different COVID-19 policies, and states implemented different restrictions and experienced different levels of compliance, so results should be expected to vary as a result of the myriad factors that affect disease transmission. As this study was limited in part by time constraints, further research is suggested into COVID-19 in the juvenile justice system within other states once data can be procured.

Conclusion

The clear racial and ethnic disparities in facility placement and sentencing support past policy knowledge and conjunctly call for further research. Texas data should be compared with other states, and research should be conducted both on youth placement and sentencing and on the support available across different racial and ethnic communities. Black youth are incarcerated more frequently than their white counterparts and as such face greater vulnerability. The COVID-19 pandemic emphasized the already-existing cycle of health disparities faced by incarcerated youth and underscored the need to break this cycle. The first step towards this is better data, which can lead to more comprehensive research and conclusions, and thus apt policy changes.

Acknowledgements

Thank you to the Break the Cycle of Children's Environmental Health Disparities program for providing this research the support to be realized. Thank you as well to the kind and helpful staff at the TJJD with whom I communicated to receive the data integral to my research. Finally, thank you to Dr. Fry for her support and feedback and for without whom this project would not have been feasible.

References

[1] Johns Hopkins Coronavirus Resource Center. URL: https://coronavirus.jhu.edu/.

[2] CDC. Health equity considerations and racial and ethnic minority groups. Centers for Disease Control and Prevention, 2021. URL: https://www.cdc.gov/coronavirus/2019-ncov/community/health-equity/race-ethnicity.html.

[3] CDC. Certain medical conditions and risk for severe COVID-19 illness. Centers for Disease Control and Prevention, 2021. URL: https://www.cdc.gov/coronavirus/2019-ncov/need-extra-precautions/people-with-medical-conditions.html.

[4] The Marshall Project. Haney declaration, 2020. URL: https://www.themarshallproject.org/documents/6884322-Haney-Declaration.

[5] American Academy of Family Physicians. Incarceration and health: A family medicine perspective (position paper). AAFP, 2017. URL: https://www.aafp.org/about/policies/all/incarceration.html.

[6] Taquet M, Geddes JR, Husain M, Luciano S, Harrison PJ. 6-month neurological and psychiatric outcomes in 236,379 survivors of COVID-19: A retrospective cohort study using electronic health records. Lancet Psychiatry 2021;8(5):416–27.

[7] Annie E Casey Foundation. Survey: Amid pandemic, youth detention population fell 24% in one month, matching a recent seven-year period. Annie E Casey Foundation, 2020. URL: https://www.aecf.org/blog/survey-amid-pandemic-youth-detention-population-fell-24-in-one-month-matchi.

[8] Hager E. Solitary, brawls, Nno teachers: Coronavirus makes juvenile jails look like adult prisons. Marshall Project, 2020. URL: https://www.themarshallproject.org/2020/05/12/solitary-brawls-no-teachers-coronavirus-makes-juvenile-jails-look-like-adult-prisons.

[9] Youth justice under the Coronavirus: Linking public health protections with the Movement for Youth Decarceration. The Sentencing Project, 2020. URL: https://www.sentencingproject.org/wp-content/uploads/2020/09/Youth-Justice-Under-the-Coronavirus.pdf.

[10] Society for Adolescent Health and Medicine. SAHM calls for action to protect justice-involved youth. AdolescentHealth.org, 2020. URL: https://www.adolescenthealth.org/About-SAHM/Press-Releases/COVID-19-Pandemic-Response-II-Calls-for-Action-to.aspx.

[11] Hager E. Many juvenile jails are now almost entirely filled with young people of color. The Marshall Project, 2021. URL: https://www.themarshallproject.org/2021/03/08/many-juvenile-jails-are-now-almost-entirely-filled-with-young-people-of-color.

[12] Office of Juvenile Justice and Delinquency Prevention. Juvenile Justice State profile: Texas. OJJDP Statistical Briefing Book. URL: https://www.ojjdp.gov/ojstatbb/special_topics/stateprofile.asp.

[13] Office of Juvenile Justice and Delinquency. Prevention COVID-19 response. URL: https://www.tjjd.texas.gov/index.php/covid19.

[14] US Census Bureau. QuickFacts. URL: https://www.census.gov/quickfacts/fact/table/US/PST045219.

[15] National Institute of Environmental Health Sciences. NIEHS COVID-19 Pandemic Vulnerability Index (PVI). US Department of Health and Human Services. URL: https://covid19pvi.niehs.nih.gov/.

[16] Office of the Texas Governor. News Press Release. URL: https://gov.texas.gov/news/category/press-release.

Chapter 3

Six month outcomes of malnourished children enrolled in the nutritional therapeutic program in a peri-urban, low-income settlement in the Western Cape, South Africa

Suzanne Kerswill*, MBChB,
Etienne Nel, PhD, FCPaed
and Thandi Wessels, FCPaed
Department of Paediatrics, University of Stellenbosch,
Department of Health - Metro East, Cape Town, South Africa

Abstract

The success of Community-based Therapeutic Care (CTC) in reducing mortality from severe acute malnutrition is well documented, although the sustainability of short-term successes is unknown. Modelled on CTC principles, the Nutrition Therapeutic Program (NTP) has been well established in the Western Cape in South Africa, but outcomes of this six-month program have yet to be measured. In this chapter we aim to determine outcomes of malnourished children after six months on the NTP, looking at weight gain, defaulting rates, and mortality, and to compare these outcomes to international sphere standards. A retrospective descriptive cohort study was conducted in a peri-urban, low-income settlement in the Western Cape. 270 patients meeting criteria for malnutrition between the age of six months and five years were recruited from three community clinics between January 2017 – December 2018. Outcomes revealed a mortality rate of 0.7%, which was

* Corresponding Author's Email: suzanneminne@gmail.com.

In: Environmental Health
Editors: I Leslie Rubin and Joav Merrick
ISBN: 979-8-88697-292-4

below the international Sphere target of <3%. Other outcomes did not meet sphere targets, with a defaulting rate of 53% (target <15%), success rate of 27% (target >75%), and average daily weight gain at six months of 0.76g/kg/day (target >3g/kg/day). We concluded that sphere targets may not be appropriate success metrics in this context, as the increased length of the program may be responsible for the higher defaulting rates, whilst recourse to in-hospital treatment means lower mortality rates are achievable. We feel that clear, achievable, and tailored local targets should be set to motivate healthcare practitioners to address the problem of childhood malnutrition in South Africa.

Introduction

The aspirational United Nations Sustainable Development Goals have envisioned a world without hunger by 2030. This challenge rings out with particular urgency in Africa, which is home to more than a third of all growth-stunted (low height/length for age) children under the age of five, and more than a quarter of all children under five with growth wasting (low weight for length/height) (1). As an upper middle-income country, South Africa should be relatively well equipped to tackle this challenge. However, it is also one of the world's most unequal societies with a Gini coefficient of 0.65 (2), and to date one third of South African children live below the food poverty line with a monthly per capita income of less than R571/41USD (2). Although progress has been made over the past decade in improving the prevalence of wasting and of self-reported hunger (2), almost a third of children under five years who die in South Africa are severely malnourished (3); and the prevalence of stunting has remained high at 27% - a figure that has not changed since 1999 (4). The recent COVID-19 outbreak has seen rising rates of hunger and food insecurity in South Africa in common with many other countries around the world (4), necessitating an effective and evidence-based response to ameliorate the impact of the pandemic on the nutritional status of our children.

The World Health Organisation (WHO) defines "severe acute malnutrition" (SAM) as a weight for height/length more than 3 z-sores below the median of the WHO growth charts, a mid-upper arm circumference less than 11.5 cm, or nutritional oedema (5). "Moderate acute malnutrition" (MAM) is defined as a weight for height/length between the -2 and -3 z-scores. "Stunting" is defined as a length/height for age below the -3 z-score (severe stunting) or between the -2 and -3 z-score (moderate stunting), and is regarded as an indicator of chronic malnutrition (6).

The cycle of childhood malnutrition

Childhood malnutrition typifies the cyclical and intergenerational nature of poverty and environmental health disparities. Malnutrition is frequently rooted antenatally, with maternal undernutrition, micronutrient deficiency, maternal illness and substance use contributing to intrauterine growth restriction, preterm labour and low birth weight (7). In infancy low breastfeeding rates, poor female education, inadequate complementary feeding, micronutrient deficiencies and infections - conditions which often prevail in poverty-stricken communities - can further contribute to childhood malnutrition (7). The period from conception to two years of life represents a critical developmental window as highlighted by UNICEF's First Thousand Days campaign (8), and intervention in this period is considered imperative in order to achieve catch-up growth (9). The sequelae of prenatal and infant malnutrition are both far-reaching and long-lasting, with detrimental effects on brain development and intelligence, earning potential, immunological function, and the incidence of non-communicable diseases in later life (8, 10, 11). The burden of malnutrition is then once again passed on to the next generation. The diagram below illustrates some of the factors that entrench the cycle of childhood malnutrition in our study setting (see Figure 1).

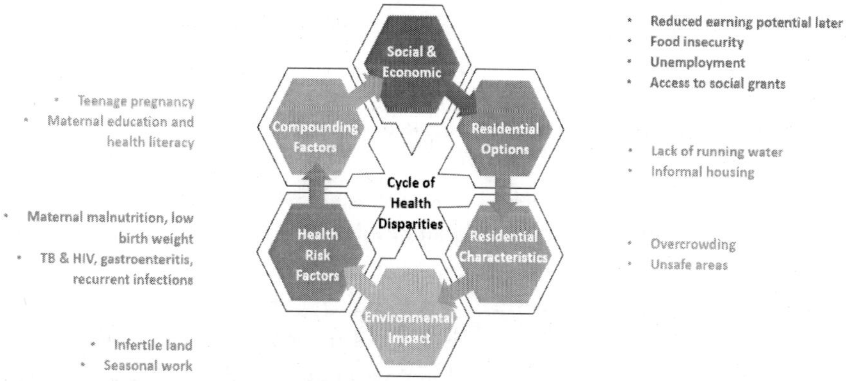

Figure 1. The cycle of poverty and child malnutrition.

How can childhood malnutrition be treated?

The complex determinants of malnutrition necessitate a unified and broad-based response to address the many structural, environmental, political, and biological underpinnings of the problem, and, clearly, no single intervention can succeed in isolation. However, over the past two decades an effective framework has been developed for the community-based treatment of acute malnutrition. Community-based Therapeutic Care (CTC) programs were developed in resource constrained settings as part of humanitarian relief efforts in Malawi, Ethiopia and Sudan where facility-based treatment for acute malnutrition was largely inaccessible (12). This framework includes a finite period of nutritional supplementation for several weeks or months, and draws on existing local resources to provide a holistic package of supportive care that is also cost effective and locally sustainable (12). These programs have demonstrated excellent early survival and recovery rates from acute malnutrition (12, 13), however little is known about the longer-term outcomes of these children.

Although early studies demonstrated that the risk of mortality following SAM is highest in the first few weeks (12), studies in other settings have shown that many deaths occur after programmatic discharge (13). The first six months post discharge emerged as a critical time-period for children with SAM in a recent systematic review looking at relapse following initial treatment (14) with lower anthropometric indices (mid-upper arm circumference and weight for height) at initial admission being the most powerful predictor of relapse in multiple studies. Furthermore, there is a need to explore the longer-term outcomes and their determinants in order to identify children at high risk and plan for a sustainable recovery. However, more information regarding the incidence and timing of adverse events is necessary in order to guide programmatic end points. Follow-up presents a further challenge, and although the WHO guideline advises that children should be monitored periodically following discharge from treatment programs to avoid relapse, follow-up has not been standardized in terms of frequency, duration, or content (15).

The efficacy of food supplementation programs beyond the setting of acute malnutrition is less well defined. A 2017 review article of community based supplementary feeding programs for food insecure, vulnerable, and malnourished populations cited a lack of consistent reporting and evidence on outcomes, particularly in the longer term (16). The review included seven Cochrane reviews and assessed the outcomes of an array of nutritional interventions in more than 12,500 malnourished or vulnerable children. The reviewers found that the effects of supplementary food interventions on growth were "modest at best", with inconsistent and limited mortality evidence. The positive impact on growth was greatest in younger children, less than two years of age, and children who are malnourished (16). A 2015 Cochrane review of food supplementation in socio-economically disadvantaged children for over six months to a year found that the effect on weight and height, although statistically significant, was small (17). The mixed and often disappointing outcomes of food supplementation programs alone as outlined above highlight the importance of a multipronged and holistic approach to tackle the root causes of malnutrition as envisioned by the CTC model.

Implementation of the CTC model

Ideally CTC programs need to be integrated into existing health care systems in order to be effective (18). This poses a considerable challenge for policy makers and health care workers alike. Due to the complex interplay of highly contextualized factors that contribute towards childhood malnutrition, local data is essential in implementing and monitoring nutritional therapeutic programs. International standards do exist to guide program monitoring, such as the Sphere Project, which outlines a set of principles and minimum humanitarian standards in technical areas of humanitarian response including nutritional interventions and treatment programs (19). The United Nations Refugee Agency (UNHCR) and World Food Program (WFP) have also suggested targets for minimum weight gain in nutritional intervention programs (15).

The 2018 Sphere targets stipulate an acceptable mortality rate of less than 3 percent for targeted supplementary feeding programs and less than 10 percent for nutritional therapeutic programs directed at children with SAM (19). The acceptable Sphere recovery rate is more than 75% and the default rate should be less than 15%. The latest edition of the Sphere Targets no longer includes a recommendation for average daily weight gain, but the UNHCR/WFP recommends a minimum average daily weight gain of 3 grams per kilogram for supplementary feeding programs and 4 grams per kilogram for therapeutic feeding programs (15).

The South African context

In South Africa, a multi-sectoral Integrated Nutrition Program was rolled out in 1994 to address malnutrition. Feeding schemes have existed as part of this program in various incarnations. In the Western Cape, the community follow-up and treatment for children with (or at risk of) malnutrition is structured within a multifaceted CTC known as the Health Facility Based Nutrition Program (20), which aims to address the underlying causes of malnutrition. Malnourished children in the Western Cape qualify for at least six months of nutritional supplementation and structured follow up as part of the Nutritional Therapeutic Program (NTP). This 6-month program represents a significantly longer period of supplementation than is described in much of the current literature - to illustrate, in one review article the mean length of stay amongst nine studies was between 40 and 50 days (12). However, the outcomes of this program remain largely unknown. Although monitoring and evaluation systems to track this intervention exist, this data is not accessible in the public domain. Moreover, the data is collated at clinic level and is not disaggregated and analyzed according to individual patient characteristics.

One small 2017 study in the Western Cape found that the mortality rate of severely malnourished children on the NTP after hospital discharge was only just within the Sphere acceptable limits at 9.5% (21). Relapse rates and loss to follow-up were not documented. Studies conducted elsewhere in South Africa (22-24) have documented extremely poor follow up rates, poor weight gain, poor documentation and problems with staff training and interpretation of growth charts.

There is still much to learn about the longer-term outcomes of CTCs, as well as the determinants of a sustainable recovery from malnutrition and the elements that contribute to programmatic success or failure. The Western Cape has a systematized, integrated NTP which is well placed to address some of these questions as it provides a relatively long-term period of nutritional supplementation and structured follow up. In light of this information, we conducted a study to describe the outcomes of malnourished children on the NTP program in our context.

Our study

The aim of this study was to describe the outcome of malnourished children enrolled in the NTP program in the Tygerberg Health Subdistrict in the Western Cape, and to identify the possible determinants of these outcomes. The outcomes of interest included mortality (during the six-month duration of the program and for a further six months thereafter), defaulting, hospital admission (up to one year after enrollment), and successful completion of the program. The definitions of "defaulters" and "treatment success" were those currently in use by the NTP: "defaulters" were defined as patients who did not attend three monthly follow-ups consecutively or who attended less than three follow-up visits overall; and treatment "success" was defined as "attaining and maintaining a normal growth curve." We also quantified the growth of participants whilst enrolled on the program in terms of absolute weight gain measured in grams per kilogram per day as well as change in z-score for weight-for-age.

The program's performance was then compared to international standards, namely the 2018 Sphere Project minimum standards for therapeutic feeding programs and targeted supplementary feeding programs and the United Nations Refugee Agency (UNHCR) and World Food Program (WFP) guidelines for minimum average daily weight gain.

Study design and setting

A retrospective descriptive cohort study was conducted to review the outcomes of patients enrolled on the NTP in a low-cost peri-urban settlement in Cape Town. This settlement was first established by the Apartheid government as an integrated service land project for people of color. Today it consists of low cost and informal housing with a high incidence of "backyard dwelling" with sub-letters erecting informal structures on existing properties. According to a 2011 census, 51% of the population in this community was under the age of 25 years (25). 51% of residents were classified as "Cape-coloured" (a multiracial ethnic group of people native to South Africa with ancestry from more than one of the various indigenous populations inhabiting the region), and 46% were black. The community has a high incidence of poverty, drug abuse, unemployment, food insecurity, challenges with service delivery, teenage pregnancy, low school completion rates, and crime leaving children at high risk of malnourishment (26, 27). Three community health clinics within a 5-kilometer radius were included in the study. All patients between the ages of six months and five years who were enrolled on the NTP program at one of these clinics between January 2017 and December 2018 for the treatment of malnutrition were included, with a resultant sample size of 270 patients. Children younger than six months and over five years of age were excluded due to problems with the definitions of moderate and severe acute malnutrition in these age-groups, and the significant contribution of perinatal complications to growth and mortality in the first six months. 39 participants (14%) had incorrect or illegible folder numbers and had to be excluded from certain sections of the analysis.

Ethics approval was obtained from the Health Research Ethics Committee of Stellenbosch University (HREC number S19/03/057), and permission to conduct the study was granted by the Tygerberg Hospital management as well as the Western Cape Department of Health (reference number WC_201905_012) and City of Cape Town (project ID 8138) health research request boards. A waiver of individual informed consent was requested as it was not feasible to contact all participants directly, and the patient data as well as clinic information was kept anonymous.

Data was collected retrospectively from the NTP registers at the participating clinics, and further information was collected using the electronic patient information platform, *Single Patient Viewer.* This platform includes a number of electronic databases, namely *Trakcare* (the National Health Laboratory Service); *Clinicom* (a hospital information management system used in the Western Cape) and *ECCR* (or "Electronic Continuity of Care Record", an online database of patient discharge summaries from public hospitals in the Western Cape). The WHO Anthro App was used to calculate anthropometric data (weight-for-age, height-for-age, and weight-for-height) from the growth parameters included in the NTP register in order to classify the nutritional status of the participants according to the WHO growth chart z-scores.

Analysis

The baseline characteristics of patients were described in terms of degree of malnutrition, age, sex, TB and HIV status and low birth weight. Overall outcomes as defined and captured by the NTP, namely death, defaulting, successful or unsuccessful completion of the program, were calculated as a percentage and compared to the Sphere targets. Weight gain during the program was described in terms of grams/kg/day as well as change in z-score for weight-for-age. Change in weight-for-height, height-for-age and mid-upper-arm circumference could not be described due to poor or inaccurate documentation. Changes in average weight-for-age over time were depicted graphically. The timing of adverse outcomes including hospitalization and defaulting were described graphically using frequency charts.

Outcomes for different exposures (low birth weight, degree of malnutrition at baseline, comorbid HIV and TB, season of enrollment, management by a nurse vs a dietitian and age) were compared in terms of average daily weight gain and change in z-score for weight-for-age over six months, as well as a poor overall outcome (defaulting, death, or unsuccessful completion). Comparative data was analyzed using univariate analysis with the appropriate statistical tests (relative risk or t-test/one way ANOVA for parametric data) using Microsoft Excel and the Statistical data analysis package.

Our findings

Table 1 summarizes the baseline characteristics of patients at enrollment. Only six patients (2%) were enrolled for SAM with the remainder being treated for "growth faltering". 146 patients (54%) were managed by a nurse, and 124 (46%) were managed by a dietitian. A very high incidence of low birth weight was noted with 37% of patients having had a low birth weight (below 2.5 kg). By comparison, the low-birth-weight rate at the nearest Midwife Obstetric Unit (primary care obstetric clinic) was 10.8% for 2017 and 11.5% for 2018 (28). The majority of children (56%) were between the age of 1 and 2 years old, with a mean age of enrollment of 2.1 years. A primary healthcare checklist had been completed for 66% of patients at enrollment. No stockouts of nutritional products were documented. Only five patients (2%) were HIV positive, but 185 (69%) had no HIV test results on trakcare. However, these patients or their mothers may have had rapid testing performed at the clinic. 19 patients (7%) were on TB treatment.

Table 1. Patient characteristics at enrollment

	n (%)
Incorrect/Illegible file number	39 (14%)
Clinic	
A	50 (19%)
B	81 (30%)
C	139 (51%)
Indication -	
Growth faltering	264 (98%)
Severe Acute Malnutrition (SAM)	6 (2%)
Managed by a nurse	146 (54%)
Managed by a dietitian	124 (46%)
Female	132 (49%)
Male	96 (36%)
Unknown (incorrect folder number)	42 (16%)
Birth Weight	
• VLBW/ELBW <1500g	20 (7%)
• LBW <2500g, >1500g	82 (30%)
• Normal >=2500g	142 (53%)
• Unknown	26 (10%)
Mean (grams)	2545
Standard deviation (grams)	631
Age at enrollment	
• Mean (years)	2,19
• Median (years)	1,86
• Infants 6 months to 1 year	44 (16%)
• 1 to 2 years	158 (56%)
• 2 to 3 years	35 (13%)
• 3 to 4 years	65 (24%)
• 4 to 5 years	32 (12%)
Primary Health Care checklist	
Complete	178 (66%)
Partial	31 (11%)
Blank	61 (23%)
Anthropometry at enrollment	
• Weight unfilled	7 (3%)
• Height unfilled	49 (18%)
• MUAC unfilled	158 (59%)

	n (%)
Stockouts at initiation	Zero
HIV lab results	
• HIV PCR positive	5 (2%)
• HIV PCR or ELISA negative	80 (30%)
• Unknown/not tested	185 (69%)
TB investigation (trakcare/single patient viewer)	
• Sputum/GW positive	10 (4%)
• Sputum/GW negative	45 (17%)
• No sputum/GW results	176 (65%)
• Unknown (incorrect fn)	39 (14%)
Number on TB treatment as per Single Patient Viewer	19 (7%)

Table 2. WHO and Wellcome Trust definitions of malnutrition

WHO definition of Severe Acute Malnutrition		
Indicator	**Measure**	**Cut-off**
Severe Wasting	Weight-for-height	< -3 standard deviations
Severe Wasting	Mid-upper-arm circumference (MUAC)	<110mm*
Bilateral Oedema	Clinical sign	

* Of note - the older (pre 2009) MUAC cut-off of <110mm is still used by the NTP implementation guidelines.

Wellcome Trust (1970) - Definition of Malnutrition		
Weight for Age (Boston centiles)	**No Oedema**	**Oedema**
60-80%	Underweight	Kwashiorkor
<60%	Marasmus	Marasmic kwashiorkor

* "SAM" as per the Wellcome Definition includes the entities of Kwashiorkor, Marasmus and Marasmic Kwashiorkor

Anthropometry

When calculating the anthropometry of participants using the indices routinely documented in the NTP register, namely weight, height/length, and mid upper arm circumference (MUAC), it became apparent that height/length and MUAC measurements were both poorly documented and, in the case of length/height, often inaccurate. A large proportion of measurements including height fell within the WHO defined "biologically implausible" range (40% of height/length-for-age and 23% of weight-for-height/length measurements - see Table 3). 18% of patients had no documented baseline height/length. MUAC was documented very infrequently, and the majority of patients (59%)

had no documented baseline MUAC. For this reason, indices including height/length or MUAC were excluded from the analysis.

The regularity and accuracy with which patient weights were documented was much better, with 97% of patients having a documented weight at baseline, and only 0.9% of weight-for-age calculations falling within the "biologically implausible" range. We therefore included only weight-for-age and average daily weight gain in the rest of the analysis.

Table 3. Comparison of nutritional status at enrollment into NTP by various measures

SECTION A: Nutritional Status at Entry into NTP according to Category Code (as captured in NTP register)	
Category Code	*n*(%)
"Growth faltering" only (1,2,8,10)	264(98%)
"SAM" (13)	6(2%)
SECTION B: Nutritional Status at Entry into NTP by Mid Upper Arm Circumference at Enrollment	
MUAC	*n*(%)
<=11.0cm	9(8%)
11-12.5cm	12(11%)
>12.5cm	91(81%)
*SAM (by WHO criteria <=11.5cm)	12(11%)
SECTION C: Z Score Anthropometry at Entry into NTP	
Weight for Age	*n*(%)
Z-score	
<=-3	60(27%)
-3 to -2	95(42%)
>-2	69(31%)
Mean (95%CI)	-2.42 (-2,57 to -2,27)
Median	-2.4
Kurtosis	2.57
Skewness	0.14
Total documented	224(83%)
Biologically Implausible Values (Flexible Exclusion Range Mean+/- 4)	
• <-6.4	1(0.4%)
• >1.6	1(0.4%)
• total	2(0.9%)

SECTION C: Z Score Anthropometry at Entry into NTP	
Height for Age	
Z-score	
<=-3	74(40%)
-3 to -2	18(10%)
>-2	92(50%)
Mean (95%CI)	-1.28 (-1.98 to -0.58)
Median	-2.1
Kurtosis	0.26
Skewness	0.71
Total documented	184(68%)
Biologically Implausible Values (Fixed Exclusion Range)	
• <-5.0	37(20%)
• >3.0	37(20%)
• total	74(40%)
Weight for Height	
Z-score	
<=-3	75(42%)
-3 to -2	14(8%)
>-2	87(49%)
Mean (95%CI)	-1.95 (-2.47 to -1.43)
Median	-2.01
Kurtosis	0.04
Skewness	0.32
Total documented	176(65%)
Biologically Implausible Values (Flexible Exclusion Range Mean +/- 4)	
• <-6.0	19(11%)
• >2.0	21(12%)
• total	40(23%)
Weight-for-Age by Age Category	**Average Z score**
6 month - 1year (*n* 39)	-2.75
1 year - 2 years (*n* 90)	-2.47
2 year -5 years (*n* 95)	-2.25
One way Anova - $F(2, 221) = 2.96$, $p = 0.05$	

Notwithstanding these problems with measurement, it was of concern that a significant number of patients with SAM may have been missed. The NTP relies on its practitioners (primarily nurses and dietitians) to classify the nutritional status of patients at enrollment (using the WHO and Wellcome definitions - see Table 2) (16). Although only six patients overall (2%) were assessed and classified as having severe acute malnutrition (SAM) at enrollment, 11% (12 patients) of those with a documented MUAC actually met the WHO definition of SAM with a MUAC below 11,5cm; and 42% (75 patients) of those with a documented weight and height/length at baseline met the criteria for SAM with a weight-for-height/length below the -3 z-score (see Table 3).

Outcomes

Table 4 depicts the main patient outcomes and compares these to the Sphere and UNHCR/WFP targets. The mortality rate was encouragingly low with only two patients (0.7%) dying from the time of enrollment to one year later. However, as out-of-facility deaths or deaths occurring outside of the Western Cape may not have been detected, the true mortality rate is likely to be as much as double the reported rate - a 2016 study in the neighbouring service area of Metro West showed that 55% of under-5 deaths occurred out of hospital (29). Even so, the true mortality rate was likely still well below the Sphere target of <10% for therapeutic feeding programs and <3% for targeted supplementary feeding programs.

Table 4. Patient outcomes and comparison to Sphere/UNHCR/WFP targets

	n (%)	**Target**
Mortality - up to 1 year after enrollment	2 (0.7%)	**SPHERE TARGET** <10% for therapeutic feeding programs (SAM) <3% for targeted supplementary feeding programs
Recovered	72 (27%) exit code "successful" • NTP definition: • once the infant/child has gained adequate weight to attain a growth curve in relation to his/her birth weight • and maintains the curve	**SPHERE TARGET** > 75% of exits from feeding program "recovered" Sphere definition: • free from medical complications • regained appetite • achieved and maintained appropriate weight gain without nutrition-related oedema (eg. for two consecutive weighings).

	n (%)	Target
Defaulted	143 (53%) "Defaulted" - i.e., failed to attend 3 consecutive visits OR "Interrupted" i.e., attended less than 3 visits in months	**SPHERE TARGET** <15%
Average Daily Weight Gain in g/kg/day (95%CI)	0.99 (95% CI 0.64 – 1.34) at 2 month follow up 0.76 (95%CI 0.60 - 0.92) at 6 months follow up	**UNHCR/WFP** guidelines for minimum average daily weight gain >3g/kg/d for supplementary feeding programs >4g/kg/d for SAM/therapeutic feeding programs (inpatient and outpatient combined)

Outcomes in terms of recovery, defaulting and average daily weight gain were below what was expected. Only 27% of patients were coded as "successful" upon completion of the 6-month program. The Sphere target for "recovery" is >75%, with recovery defined as "being free from medical complications, having regained appetite and having achieved and maintained appropriate weight gain without nutrition-related oedema (e.g., for two consecutive weighings)."

The defaulting rate was 53% with a Sphere target of <15%. Although this defaulting rate is well above target, it should be noted that the NTP program is significantly longer than most therapeutic feeding programs cited in the literature. However, more than 20% of patients never returned for follow-up after being enrolled. Overall, almost half of patients did attend at least 3 follow-up visits.

The average daily weight gain was below target at 0.99 grams per kilogram per day (95% CI 0.64 - 1.34) at 2 months and 0.76 grams per kilogram per day (95%CI 0.60 - 0.92) at 6 months follow up, with a UNHCR/WFP target of at least 3g/kg/day for supplementary feeding programs and 4g/kg/day for therapeutic feeding programs targeting severe malnutrition.

We reviewed the timing of admission to hospital and defaulting - see Figure 3. Patients were particularly vulnerable to illness requiring hospitalization in the first four months after enrollment, with a total number of admissions greater than 10 per month for this period. The most common reasons for admission were for respiratory illness (62%), diarrheal disease (11%), and nutritional problems (6%). There was a small late peak of admissions at nine months (with a total of seven admissions), but admission rates remained very low thereafter up until one year post admission or six months post completion of the NTP. A progressive attrition in clinic attendance was noted during the six months on the program (see Figure 4). The reasons for this need to be explored in future research. One small qualitative study elsewhere in Cape Town which explored the perspectives of mothers of children on the NTP found that although most mothers expressed satisfaction with receiving the supplements, they had felt they had received little or no education, and many mothers had experienced "poor communication with staff members as well as unfavourable comments and lack of respect." (30)

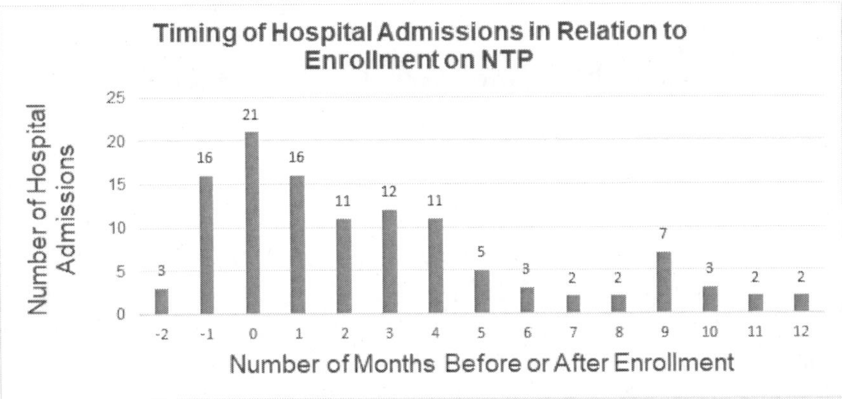

Figure 3. Timing of adverse events.

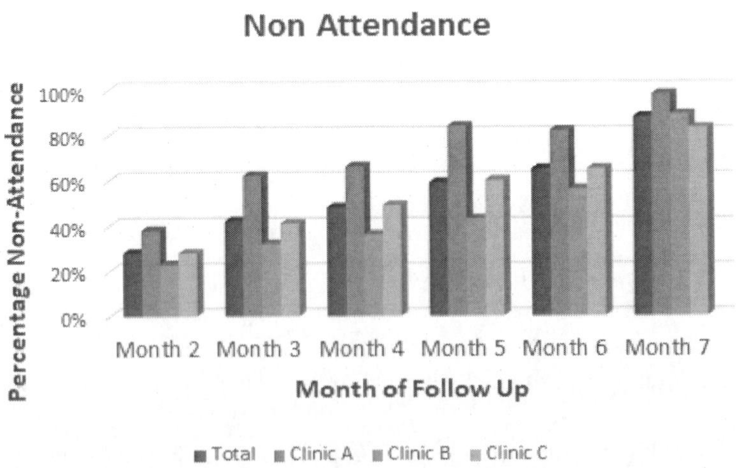

Figure 4. Timing of adverse events.

Associations between clinical, social, and programmatic determinants and outcome at six months

The total growth of participants over six months was measured (in grams per kilogram per day as well as change in z-score for weight-for-age), and associations were sought between weight gain and potential determinants as described elsewhere (14) – see Table 5.

Younger infants were found to have better weight gain when compared with older children. The average weight gain in infants aged six months to one year was 1,18g/kg/day (95% CI 0.97 to 1.38), compared with 0.87g/kg/day (95% CI 0.66 to 1,07) in infants aged 1-2 years, and only 0.46g/kg/day (95% CI 0.17 to 0.76) in older children aged 2-5 years ($p = 0.002$). Although this was unsurprising given the greater growth velocity expected in younger children, average increases in weight-for-age were also greater for younger children which would be unaffected by differences in expected growth velocity. For example, the average increase in weight-for-age z-score for infants 1-2 years old was 0.52 (95%CI 0.15 to 0.88); whereas older children aged 2-5 years displayed an average drop in z-score after six months of 0,06 (95%CI -0.52 to 0,40). However, this result did not reach statistical significance ($p = 0.07$). These findings are in keeping with other studies (17) which have demonstrated greater weight gain in younger infants.

The season of enrollment also emerged as a possible predictor of outcome, with children enrolled in the summer or autumn months faring better than those enrolled in winter or spring in terms of total weight gain. The reasons for this are unknown and need further research, but may reflect seasonal changes in diet or household income (caregivers may be employed locally as farm labourers). Children enrolled from December to May demonstrated an average increase in z-score for weight-for-age over six months of 0.52 (95%CI 0.22 to 0.82) whilst those enrolled between June and November showed no significant change in z score (average 0.01; 95%CI - 0.37 to 0.39). When compared using a t-test these values were significantly different (p- 0.03). Total weight gain in terms of grams per kilogram per day showed a similar pattern, with an average increase of 0.89 g/kg/day (95%CI 0.74 to 1.04) during summer/autumn and only 0.62 g/kg/day (95%CI 0.34 to 0.91) during winter/spring. However, the t-test p-Value of 0.10 was not statistically significant here.

Table 5. Factors associated with weight gain at six months follow-up

	n(%)	Average weight gain in g/kg/day (95%CI)	Test statistic	*n*(%)	Average change in weight for age Z-score (95%CI)	Test statistic
Sex			Independent t-test (unequal variance) p-Value 0.32			Independent t-test (unequal variance) Two-tail t-test p-value 0.18
Female	50(66%)	0.84 (0.68 to 1.0)		47(65%)	0.43 (0.21 to 0.65)	
Male	26(34%)	0.70 (0.49 to 0.68)		25(35%)	0.02 (-0.54 to 0.59)	
Age			One-way ANOVA p-Value 0.002			One-way ANOVA p-Value 0.07
6months-1yr	19(21%)	1.18 (0.97 to 1.38)		15(21%)	0.49 (0.20 to 0.79)	
1-2 years	34(37%)	0.87 (0.66 to 1.07)		29(40%)	0.52 (0.15 to 0.88)	
2-5years	38(42%)	0.46 (0.17 to 0.76)		28(39%)	-0.06 (-0.52 to 0.40)	
TB Status			Independent t-test (Unequal variances) p-Value 0.86			Independent t-test (Unequal variances) p-Value 0.80
Positive	7(9%)	0.79 (0.13 to 1.44)		5(7%)	0.36 (-0.74 to 1.45)	
Negative	70(11%)	0.73 (0.54 to 0.93)		67(93%)	0.25 (-0.01 to 0.51)	
HIV Status			Independent t-test (Unequal variance) p-Value 0.16			Independent t-test (Unequal variances) p-Value 0.39
Positive	3(4%)	1.13 (-0.11 to 2.36)		3(4%)	0.68 (-0.97 to 2.34)	
Negative	74(96%)	0.72 (0.54 to 0.91)		69(96%)	0.24 (-0.01 to 0.49)	

	n(%)	**Average weight gain in g/kg/day (95%CI)**	**Test statistic**	*n*(%)	**Average change in weight for age Z-score (95%CI)**	**Test statistic**
Baseline MUAC						
<=11cm	4(11%)	0.78 (-0.46 to 2.04)	Anova	3(10%)	-0.18 (-3.59 to 3.24)	Anova
11 - 12,5cm	11(30%)	1.05 (0.51 to 1.58)	p-value 0.37	3(13%)	0.56 (-4.49 to 5.62)	p-Value 0.81
>12,5cm	22(59%)	0.51 (0.00 to 1.02)		23(77%)	0.17 (-0.32 to 0.65)	
Baseline Z-score for Weight for Height (implausible values excluded)						
<-2	31(63%)	1.01 (0.78 to 1.24)	Two tailed t-test p-value 0.01	32(65%)	0.62 (0.29 to 0.95)	Two tailed t-test p-value 0.03
=>-2	18(37%)	0.62 (0.44 to 0.81)		17(35%)	0.17 (-0.07 to 0.4)	
Baseline Z-score Height for Age (implausible values excluded)						
<=-2	19(51%)	0.67 (0.47 to 0.86)	Two-tailed t-test P-value 0.08	18(50%)	0.25 (-0.02 to 0.51)	Two tailed t-test P-Value 0.32
>-2	18(49%)	0.94 (0.68 to 1.2)		18(50%)	0.48 (0.07 to 0.88)	

Table 5. (Continued)

	n(%)	Average weight gain in g/kg/day (95%CI)	Test statistic	*n*(%)	Average change in weight for age Z-score (95%CI)	Test statistic
Baseline z score Weight for Age						
<=-3	18(24%)	0.86 (0.62 to 1.10)	Anova	18(25%)	0.40 (0.10 to 0.70)	Anova p-Value 0.10
-3 to -2	30(41%)	0.87 (0.64 to 1.10)	p-Value 0.21	28(39%)	0.53 (0.16 to 0.89)	
>-2	26(35%)	0.52 (0.07 to 0.97)		26(36%)	-0.05 (0.55 to 0.46)	
Number of Follow-ups						
<=4fups	19(21%)	0.57 (-0.07 to 1.19)	Anova	15(20%)	0.41(-0.37 to 1.19)	Anova p-Value 0.14
5 fups	52(57%)	0.87 (0.71 to 1.03)	p-Value 0.27	42(55%)	0.88 (0.69 to 1.08)	
6 fup	21(23%)	0.69 (0.52 to 0.85)		19(25%)	0.67 (0.50 to 0.84)	
Ex Low Birth Weight						
<2500g	38(41%)	0.85 (0.68 to 1.01)	Independent t-test (unequal variance)	31(42%)	0.34 (-0.04 to 0.71)	Independent t-test (unequal variance)
>=2500g	54(59%)	0.70 (0.46 to 0.95)	Two-tailed t-test p-Value 0.34	42(58%)	0.21 (-0.12 to 0.54)	Two-tailed t-test P-value 0.61

	n(%)	**Average weight gain in g/kg/day (95%CI)**	**Test statistic**	*n*(%)	**Average change in weight for age Z-score (95%CI)**	**Test statistic**
Nurse vs Dietitian						
Nurse	40(43%)	0.71 (0.38 to 1.05)	Independent t-test Unequal variance)	35(48%)	0.20 (-0.28 to 0.68)	Independent t-test unequal variance)
Dietitian	52(57%)	0.80 (0.68 to 0.92)	Two-tailed t-test P-value 0.62	38(52%)	0.32 (0.15 to 0.50)	Two-tailed t-test P-value 0.64
Season of enrollment						
Summer/Autumn (Dec - May)	49(53%)	0.89 (0.74 to 1.04)	Two-tailed t-test (unequal variance) p-Value 0.10	38(52%)	0.52 (0.22 to 0.82)	Two-tailed t-test (unequal variance) p-Value 0.03
Winter/Spring (June- Nov)	43(47%)	0.62 (0.34 to 0 91)		35(48%)	-0.01 (-0.39 to 0.37)	

The last factors that yielded a statistically significant association with total weight gain were the degree of stunting and of wasting at baseline. However, the high rates of measurement error of height outlined in the section on baseline anthropometry made the interpretation of these results difficult. "Biologically implausible values" as defined in the section on baseline anthropometry were excluded from the final analysis in order to remove the likelihood of obvious errors from the calculation.

A small but statistically significant difference in weight gain was found in patients with wasting versus no wasting at baseline. Children with severe or moderate wasting achieved almost double the weight gain of their counterparts with no wasting at baseline, with an average daily weight gain of 1.01g/kg/day (95%CI 0.78 to 1.24) versus 0.62g/kg/day (95%CI 0.44 to 0.81; *p*- 0,01.) Similarly, children with wasting at baseline achieved greater improvements in z-score for weight-for-age over the 6 months: their z-scores increased by an average of 0.62 (95%CI 0.29 to 0.95) versus 0.17 (95%CI -0.07 to 0.4) in those with no wasting, *p*- 0.03.

Conversely, participants with severe stunting at baseline achieved only around two thirds of the daily weight gain attained by those with no stunting, with an average daily weight gain of 0.67g/kg/day (95%CI 0.47 to 0.86) compared to 0.94g/kg/day (95%CI 0.68 to 1.2). However, these values were not statistically significant (*p*-Value of 0.08). This is possibly due to the small sample size of 37 patients resulting from a large proportion of missing or excluded data. Once again, the high levels of measurement error of height also need to be taken into consideration here.

No significant association was found between a number of other possible predictors (namely sex, TB disease, HIV status, baseline MUAC, baseline weight-for-age z-score, number of follow-ups, low birth weight, or dietitian versus nurse administered NTP) and weight gain over 6 months in terms of average daily weight gain or change in z-scores for weight-for-age. Small sample sizes for some of these factors (including HIV and TB positive patients and baseline MUAC) limited the interpretation of these findings.

A correlation was sought between a number of possible determinants and a poor overall outcome as defined by any NTP exit code other than "successful". This included defaulters, interrupters, deaths and patients coded as "unsuccessful". Patients who did not default but had no documented exit code were excluded from the analysis. A positive HIV status was associated with a small increased relative risk (1.37; 95%CI 1.28-1.48) of an adverse outcome. Patients who were managed by a nurse had an increased relative risk of a poor outcome of 1.56 (95%CI 1.30-1.87) when compared with patients who were managed by a dietitian. No relationship was found between a poor overall outcome and TB status, low birth weight, hospital admission (at any point from two months prior to one year post enrollment on the NTP), or an incomplete Primary Health Care checklist at admission (includes deworming, immunization status, TB screening, Vit A up to date).

Table 6. Relative risk of poor outcome (defaulting/unsuccessful/deaths) for different exposures

	n(%)	Relative Risk/95%CI	p-Value
HIV Status			
Positive	5(2%)	1.37 (1.28-1.48)	<0.0001
Negative	265(98%)		
TB Status			
Positive	18(7%)	1.06 (0.82-1.38)	0.63
Negative	252(93%)		
Low birth weight <2500g			
Yes	73(38%)	1.00 (0.81-1.23)	0.98
No	121(62%)		
Hospital admission (2months pre to 1 year post enrollment)			
Yes	40(18%)	1.15 (0.93 -1.41)	0.19
No	178(82%)		
Primary Health Care Completed at enrollment			
Yes	140(64%)	1.21 (0.98 - 1.5)	0.08
No	78((36%)		
Nurse vs Dietitian administered			
Nurse	88(40%)	1.56 (1.30-1.87)	<0.0001
Dietitian	130(60%)		

Discussion

At first glance, the implementation of the NTP is performing well in this setting in terms of mortality, but poorly in terms of recovery, adherence and weight gain when compared to the Sphere and UNHCR/WFP targets. However, the definition of "success" needs to be examined in greater detail. At present no clear local targets are stipulated in terms of the programmatic aims, and the international Sphere and UNHCR/WFP targets may not be an appropriate benchmark in this setting. Firstly, given the six-month long duration of the program, a defaulting target of less than 15% may be too stringent. Higher follow-up rates are much more attainable over shorter periods, whereas some degree of loss-to-follow-up over much longer treatment periods are probably to be expected. Nonetheless, efforts should be made to explore the reasons for loss to follow-up and to improve treatment adherence. With the recent strengthening of community-based care workers in Cape Town, active case finding and follow-up of patients who have defaulted in their homes should be prioritized.

Secondly, although the low mortality rate is encouraging, it is perhaps unsurprising given the relatively good access to resources such as hospital admission in this setting. A lower target for mortality would likely be appropriate and achievable. Lastly, the definitions of "treatment success" need further clarification. Definitions for "nutritional recovery" have varied, but most - including the definition used in the Sphere targets - have been used to refer to recovery from SAM and as such include clinical criteria such as return of appetite and the resolution of nutritional oedema (19). The definition used by the NTP of "attaining and maintaining an adequate growth curve in relation to his/her growth curve" is perhaps more suited to the setting of moderate acute as well as chronic malnutrition. However, this definition relies heavily on clinic practitioners to interpret growth curves, and therefore lacks objectivity. It also focuses only on the measurement of weight-for-age and not length/height-for-age (a better marker of chronic malnutrition), or MUAC (15). This problematic emphasis is reflected in the poor documentation of length/height and MUAC. At present, the measurement of height/length was found to be inaccurate, and the MUAC was documented infrequently. This could result in the misclassification of the nutritional status of children with significant consequences, such as having patients who qualify for treatment being denied access to the NTP program or missing instances of SAM requiring urgent treatment.

It is critical that clear local targets are set in order to guide the implementation of the NTP and to keep clinic practitioners accountable and motivated. These targets need to address the current status of childhood malnutrition in South Africa. As a bundle of care, the NTP is being used to treat a broad spectrum of nutritional problems ranging from uncomplicated moderate and severe acute malnutrition with its attendant risk of immune compromise, comorbid infection and even death; to chronic malnutrition in the form of stunting, which should ideally be treated aggressively in the first two years of life in order to avoid long term losses in growth and intellectual potential. Furthermore, as demonstrated in this study, intervention seems to be most effective in the first two years of life in terms of achieving the greatest weight gain. Clear targets need to be set for different groups of children (acutely malnourished children with growth wasting and chronically malnourished children with growth stunting), with an emphasis on initiating treatment within the first two years of life. The success of any nutritional intervention also relies on its ability to detect malnutrition early, and as such targets for community screening need to be set and routinely measured.

Other areas of programmatic implementation that require attention include the poor and inaccurate documentation of height and MUAC (demanding regular staff training, equipment checks and targets for completion rates); mechanisms for tracing the 20% of patients who fail to return after being initiated on treatment; and clear targets for the interventions that are likely to empower patients and achieve a more sustainable recovery, including linkages with other community resources and high-quality dietary counselling. The fact that management by a dietitian versus a nurse was protective against a poor outcome reinforces the value of nutritional counselling. Where the program is delivered by nurses, further training and standardization in the content of nutritional counselling may be of benefit. Both the content and the delivery of nutritional counselling are likely to be important, as a qualitative study elsewhere in Cape Town found that mothers experienced poor communication, a lack of education and a perceived lack of respect (30) which may be a contributing factor to the high defaulting rates. Regardless of which healthcare professional administers the NTP it is critical that the counselling received is practical and evidence-based and that it is delivered in an empathetic and empowering manner.

The poor weight gain achieved by patients in this study is of concern. A number of possible explanations exist. Firstly, the phenomenon of sharing of nutritional supplements to other family members in food insecure households is a well described and understandable phenomenon (17). This reinforces the importance of a holistic approach and of appropriate patient referral to other resources (such as community-based workers and assistance in accessing social grants). Secondly, although the defaulting rates were better than have been reported elsewhere in South Africa (24), attendance was inconsistent and a progressive attrition in follow-up was noted over the course of 6 months. The reasons for this need further exploration. Importantly, not all groups of patients gained weight equally. In this study, younger patients and patients with more severe wasting at baseline tended to demonstrate better weight gain, which is in keeping with findings elsewhere (16). On the other hand, patients with stunting at baseline tended to achieve less weight gain. Taken together with the long-term neurodevelopmental consequences of childhood stunting (11), this vulnerable group demands particular care and attention.

Although a number of problems and challenges have been discussed above, the NTP also has many potential strengths. This large-scale program was well integrated into the routine functioning of these clinics, and all of the NTP registers were readily available and up to date. A total of 537 patient visits were recorded for the 270 patients over the course of two years. Documentation of certain parameters was excellent – 90% of patients had a documented birth weight and 97% had a documented weight at enrollment. 98% of the 94 patients who attended follow-up at six months had a documented exit weight. The primary healthcare checklist had been completed in full for 66% of patients and in part for 11% of patients, showing that the majority of malnourished patients received a package of basic medical care. Unlike in other studies elsewhere in South Africa, stockouts of nutritional products did not appear to be a problem. These strengths need to be harnessed and built upon in order to fully realize the potential of this program as a nutritional intervention and data source to improve our understanding of the long-term treatment, outcomes and effects of malnutrition.

The current NTP implementation guidelines for the Western Cape are due to be revised in the near future, and by including a number of key changes the programme could be strengthened significantly.

Treatment duration

Due to its longer duration of six months, the NTP is well placed to address the uncertainty that remains around the optimal treatment duration of acute malnutrition. In this study, there was a higher incidence of admission to hospital in the first four months as well as a smaller peak of hospital admissions at nine months (three months after completion of the program). This suggests that children remain immunologically compromised secondary to malnutrition and are vulnerable to infection for the first four months on the programme, with the majority of admissions being for respiratory or diarrhoeal illness. Although weight gain was poor overall, the best weight gain was demonstrated in the first four months of treatment. We were unable to assess the risk of relapse as we did not have access to patient anthropometry after discharge from the program. Of note, a significant risk of late relapse has been reported elsewhere (14). There was no late mortality in the six months following discharge from the program. Based on this information, a treatment duration of at least four months would seem beneficial. However, a case-control study would be ideal to address this question more robustly. A routine follow-up several months following discharge from the program could be instituted in order to identify treatment relapse and to evaluate the longer-term impact of the program. Strategies to prevent defaulting and trace treatment defaulters need to be developed.

Limitations

The retrospective design of this study and the lack of a control group limited its utility in fully assessing the impact of the NTP on childhood growth. A prospective case control study is recommended in future to further explore some of our findings. The poor documentation of height and MUAC were important findings in this study, but unfortunately this also meant that we were unable to comment meaningfully on growth parameters including these indices and had to rely heavily on parameters including only weight (i.e., weight-for-age and average daily weight gain).

Conclusion

When compared to the international Sphere and UNHCR/WFP targets, the NTP performed well in this setting in terms of mortality, but poorly in terms of treatment success, defaulting and growth. However, it is debatable whether these targets are an appropriate benchmark in our context. Local targets need to be clearly stipulated and calibrated to the South African context of a persistently high burden of chronic malnutrition and stunting, as well as the unfolding fallout of the COVID 19 pandemic and fear of the disease with rising unemployment, poverty, and food insecurity.

The NTP in the Western Cape is an example of a well-integrated model of care for malnourished children based on the CTC model. Although many challenges with the implementation and monitoring of such a large-scale program exist as outlined above, this program has significant potential in interrupting the cycle of childhood malnutrition at multiple levels as illustrated below. Although we have attempted to measure the tangible outcomes of a program to treat malnutrition, we acknowledge that many inputs into the health and wellbeing of these children are impossible to measure and we wish to recognise the hard work and dedication of the healthcare workers and administrators who have helped to implement this program and to interrupt the legacy of childhood malnutrition (see Figure 2).

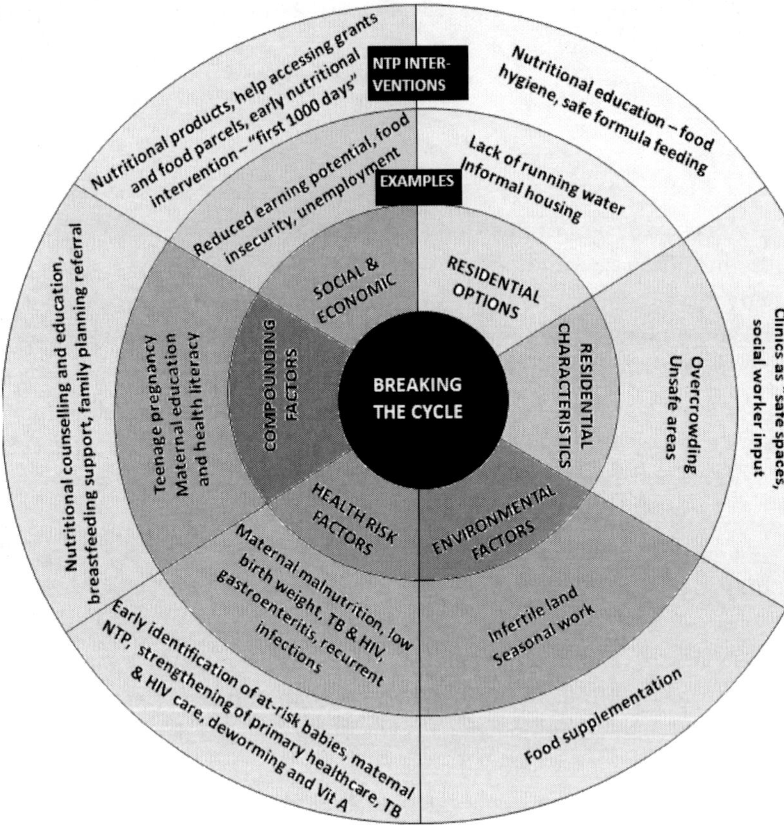

Figure 2. Strategies to break the cycle of poverty and child malnutrition.

Acknowledgements

The author extends grateful acknowledgement to the following persons for their insights and assistance with this study: Joy Williams, Community Dietitian; Tanja Venter, Community Dietitian and Michael McCaul, Researcher/Biostatistian.

References

[1] Mathers C, Boerma T, Hogan D, Ho J, Retno Mahanani, Emi Suzuki W, Gerland P, et al. Levels and trends in child mortality. UN Inter-agency Group for Child Mortality Estimation. World Bank Document, 2017. URL: http://documents1.worldbank.org/curated/en/358381508420391876/pdf/120551-REVISED-PUBLIC-IGME-report-2017-child-mortality-final.pdf.

[2] UNICEF Malnutrition in Children - UNICEF data 2020. URL: https://data.unicef.org/topic/nutrition/malnutrition/.

[3] Bamford LJ, Mckerrow NH, Barron P, Aung Y. Child mortality in South Africa: Fewer deaths, but better data are needed. S Afr Med J 2018;108(3 Suppl 1):S25–32.

[4] Haddad L. Foreword. In: May J, Witten C, Lake L, eds. South African Child Gauge 2020. Cape Town: Children's Institute, University of Cape Town, 2020.

[5] UNHCR/WFP. UNHCR/WFP Guidelines for selective feeding: The management of malnutrition in emergencies, 2011. URL: https://www.unhcr.org/publications/operations/4b7421fd20/guidelines-selective-feeding-management-malnutrition-emergencies.html.

[6] Collins S. Treating severe acute malnutrition seriously. Arch Dis Child 2007;92(5):453-461. doi:10.1136/adc.2006.098327.

[7] Allen L, Gillespie S. What works? A review of the efficacy and effectiveness of nutrition interventions. UN-ACC/SCN Nutrition policy paper 2001. URL: https://www.researchgate.net/publication/228377212_What_Works_A_Review_of_the_Efficacy_and_Effectiveness_of_Nutrition_Interventions/citation/download.

[8] UNICEF. Cusick S, Georgieff MK. The first 1,000 days of life: The brain's window of opportunity. URL: https://www.unicef-irc.org/article/958-the-first-1000-days-of-life-the-brains-window-of-opportunity.html.

[9] Prentice AM, Ward KA, Goldberg GR, Jarjou LM, Moore SE, Fulford AJ, et al. Critical windows for nutritional interventions against stunting. Am J Clin Nutr 2013;97(5):911–8. doi.org/10.3945/ajcn.112.052332.

[10] Lelijveld N, Seal A, Wells JC, Kirkby J, Opondo C, Chimwezi E, et al. Chronic disease outcomes after severe acute malnutrition in Malawian children (ChroSAM): A cohort study. Lancet Global Health 2016;4(9):e654–62.

[11] Prendergast AJ, Humphrey JH. The stunting syndrome in developing countries. Paediatr Int Child Health 2014;34(4):250–65.

[12] Collins S, Sadler K, Dent N, Khara T, Guerrero S, Myatt M, et al. Key issues in the success of community-based management of severe malnutrition. Food Nutr Bull 2006;27(Suppl 3):S49–82.

[13] Kerac M, Bunn J, Chagaluka G, Bahwere P, Tomkins A, Collins S, et al. Follow-up of post-discharge growth and mortality after treatment for severe acute

malnutrition (FuSAM study): A prospective cohort study. PLoS One 2014; 9(6):e96030.

[14] Stobaugh HC, Mayberry A, McGrath M, Bahwere P, Zagre NM, Manary MJ, et al. Relapse after severe acute malnutrition: A systematic literature review and secondary data analysis. Matern Child Nutr 2019;15(2):e12702.

[15] UNHCR/WFP. UNHCR/WFP Guidelines for selective feeding: The management of malnutrition in emergencies, 2011. URL: https://www.unhcr.org/publications/operations/4b7421fd20/guidelines-selective-feeding-management-malnutrition-emergencies.html.

[16] Visser J, Mclachlan MH, Maayan N, Garner P. Community-based supplementary feeding for food insecure, vulnerable and malnourished populations: An overview of systematic reviews. Cochrane Database Syst Rev 2018;11(11):CD010578.

[17] Kristjansson E, Francis DK, Liberato S, Benkhalti Jandu M, Welch V, Batal M, et al. Food supplementation for improving the physical and psychosocial health of socio-economically disadvantaged children aged three months to five years Cochrane Database Syst Rev 2015;2015(3):CD009924.

[18] Collins S. Treating severe acute malnutrition seriously. Arch Dis Child. 2007;92(5):453-461. doi.org/10.1136/adc.2006.098327.

[19] Sphere Association. The Sphere handbook: Humanitarian charter and minimum standards in humanitarian response, fourth edition. Geneva: Sphere Association, 2018. URL: http://www.spherestandards.org/handbook.

[20] Western Cape Department of Health. Policy and implementation guidelines for the Nutrition Supplementation Programme of the Health Facility Based Nutrition Programme (HFBNP). Cape Town: Western Cape Provincial Government, 2011.

[21] Groenewald M, Jenkins L. Evaluating the growth, associated co-morbidities and mortality in children under the age of five years, six months after treatment for severe acute malnutrition (SAM) in the Oudtshoorn sub-district. Stellenbosch: Stellenbosch University, 2017. URL: https://scholar.sun.ac.za.

[22] Brits H, Joubert G, Eyman K, de Vink R, Lesaoana K, Makhetha S, et al. An assessment of the integrated nutrition programme for malnourished children aged six months to five years at primary healthcare facilities in Mangaung, Free State, South Africa. AJOL 2017;59(6):214–8. URL: https://www.ajol.info/index.php/safp/article/view/163991.

[23] Selvaggio P, Selvaggio MP, Goldman I. Western Cape province case study report. Diagnostic/implementation evaluation of nutrition interventions for children from conception to age 5, 2014. URL: https://evaluations.dpme.gov.za/evaluations/441/documents/4536a5f1-9538-43b9-9d48-71eb5f4d7234.

[24] Hendricks M, le Roux M, Fernandes M, Irlam J. Evaluation of a nutrition supplementation programme in the Northern Cape Province of South Africa. Public Health Nutr 2003;6(5):431–7.

[25] Statistics South Africa. Statistical release. Census 2011. Pretoria, 2012. URL: http://www.statssa.gov.za/publications/p03014/p030142011.pdf.

[26] Gie J. Crime in Cape Town: 2001-2008. Cape Town: GCIS, 2009. URL: https://citeseerx.ist.psu.edu/viewdoc/download?doi=10.1.1.560.9602&rep=rep1&type=pdf.

[27] Watt MH, Meade CS, Kimani S, MacFarlane JC, Choi KW, Skinner D, et al. The impact of methamphetamine ("tik") on a peri-urban community in Cape Town, South Africa. Int J Drug Polic. 2014;25(2):219-25.

[28] Unpublished data from the Perinatal Problem Identification Program – PIPP. Communicated by Dr Y Prinsloo, 2021.

[29] Reid AE, Hendricks MK, Groenewald P, Bradshaw D. Where do children die and what are the causes? Under-5 deaths in the Metro West geographical service area of the Western Cape, South Africa, 2011. S Afr Med J 2016;106(4):359–64.

[30] Andresen EC, Wandel M, Eide WB, Herselman M, Iversen PO. Delivery of the Nutrition Supplementation Programme in the Cape Town metropolitan area from the perspective of mothers of under-5s: A qualitative study. SAJCH 2009;3(3):90–5.

Chapter 4

Does early life phthalate exposure mediate racial disparities in children's cognitive abilities?

Marisa A Patti[1,*], MHS, Melissa Eliot[1], PhD, Nan Li[1], PhD, Kimberly Yolton[2], PhD, Bruce P Lanphear[3,4], MPH, MD, Aimin Chen[5], MD, PhD and Joseph M Braun[1], RN, MSPH, PhD

[1]Department of Epidemiology, Brown University, Providence, Rhode Island, United States of America

[2]Department of Pediatrics, Division of General and Community Pediatrics, Cincinnati Children's Hospital Medical Center, University of Cincinnati College of Medicine, Cincinnati, Ohio, United States of America

[3]Child and Family Research Institute, British Columbia Children's Hospital, Vancouver, British Columbia, Canada

[4]Faculty of Health Sciences, Simon Fraser University, Burnaby, British Columbia, Canada

[5]Department of Biostatistics, Epidemiology and Informatics, University of Pennsylvania, Philadelphia, Pennsylvania, United States of America

Abstract

Exposure to phthalates is associated with diminished cognition. It is unknown, however, if disproportionate exposure to phthalates among racial minorities contributes to racial disparities in children's intellectual abilities. *Methods*: We used data from 253 mother-child pairs in Cincinnati, OH (HOME Study, 2003-2006). We measured urinary concentrations of eleven phthalate metabolites twice during pregnancy

---

* *Correspondence:* Marisa A Patti, MHS, Doctoral Candidate, Department of Epidemiology, The Brown University School of Public Health, Providence, Rhode Island and 120 W 21st Street, Apt 511 New York, NY 10011, United States. Email: marisapatti@gmail.com.

and up to six times in childhood. We evaluated children's cognitive abilities at ages 5 and 8 years. Using causal mediation models, we quantified covariate-adjusted direct and indirect effects of race on children's Full Scale IQ scores for individual phthalate metabolite concentrations during gestation and childhood. *Results*: Average IQ scores among Black children (n=90) were 7.0-points lower (95% CI: -12, -1.8) than White children (n=145) after adjustment for socioeconomic factors. Urinary monobenzyl phthalate (MBzP) and monoethyl phthalate (MEP) concentrations during gestation and childhood were higher among Black children. We did not observe compelling evidence that phthalate mediated the race-IQ association, with the exception of MEP. Childhood MEP concentrations partially mediated the race-IQ association. For instance, the disparities in IQ scores between Black and White children would have been reduced by 1.9 points (95% CI: -4.7, 0.7) for each 10-fold reduction in urinary MEP concentrations at age 2 years. Other phthalate metabolite concentrations during pregnancy or childhood did not mediate the race-IQ association. Conclusions: We found that urinary MEP concentrations partly mediated IQ disparities among HOME Study children. Reducing exposure to some phthalates might help reduce IQ disparities among Black and White children.

Introduction

Phthalates are a class of chemicals used in personal care and consumer products including some cosmetics, pharmaceuticals, vinyl flooring, medical supplies, food packaging, and plastic toys (1–7). Given the wide range of phthalate containing products, human exposure can occur through dermal absorption, inhalation, or ingestion (1, 4, 8). While phthalates are quickly excreted from the body (<24 hours), exposure is often chronic and ubiquitous in the US population, including among vulnerable sub-populations like pregnant women, infants, and children (3, 9). Exposure may be higher in infants and children than adults due to differences physiology, diet, and behaviors (e.g., mouthing) (9–14).

Phthalates are also suspected developmental neurotoxicants (15–23). Indeed some, but not all epidemiologic studies (24, 25) report an inverse association of gestational (17–22) or childhood exposure (16, 18–20) to some phthalates with child cognitive abilities (i.e., Intelligence Quotient [IQ]). While measures of intelligence are imperfect and at times controversial, they are strong predictors of educational achievement and work performance (26–30). Racial disparities in child IQ have been previously documented in the US and abroad, such that some racial and ethnic minorities tend to have lower IQ measures relative to their White peers (31–33). Genetics do not explain the full heterogeneity in child IQ, (34, 35) emphasizing the need to consider external factors such as environmental exposures and socioeconomic features (36). Further, race is a social construct, not a biological variable. No genetic basis exists to explain racial disparities in IQ, indicating that disparities in cognitive abilities are most likely are related to social, economic and environmental factors (31, 33, 37).

While phthalate exposure is nearly universal in the United States (US), exposure to some phthalates are consistently higher amongst non-White racial groups, (13, 38) particularly Blacks (9, 39, 40). Moreover, prior work has attributed racial and ethnic disparities in reproductive and cardiometabolic health outcomes to racial and ethnic differences in phthalate exposure (13, 38, 40–42). This highlights how certain subsets of the population may be more heavily exposed and vulnerable to the adverse effects of environmental toxicants, including phthalates (43). Despite the recognition that racial and ethnic differences exist in phthalate exposure and child IQ, no study has evaluated whether increased phthalate exposure among non-Hispanic Black children mediates the relation between race and child IQ.

Using data from the Health Outcomes and Measures of the Environment (HOME) Study, we first quantified racial disparities in gestational and childhood phthalate exposure, as well as child IQ. Second, we assessed if phthalates mediate the relation between race and child IQ to determine if disparities in child cognition could be attributed, in part, to phthalate exposure (44). While this study focused on phthalates, it also served a proof-of-principle analysis of environmental toxicants as some possible explanatory factors of racial disparities in child IQ.

Our study

The HOME Study is a general population, prospective pregnancy and birth cohort study. Information regarding recruitment and data collection details have been previously published (45). Briefly, we recruited 468 pregnant women from 1,263 eligible women from nine prenatal clinics affiliated with three delivery hospitals in the greater Cincinnati, Ohio area between 2003 and 2006. Inclusion criteria specified women be at least 18 years old, 16±3 weeks gestation, HIV-negative, not taking medications for seizures and/or thyroid disorders and living in homes built before 1978, and not having a diagnosis of diabetes, bipolar disorder, schizophrenia, or cancer that resulted in radiation treatment or chemotherapy. The Institutional Review Board at Cincinnati Children's Hospital Medical Center and all participating hospitals approved this study. All participants provided their written, informed consent for themselves and their children.

Of 468 women who enrolled, 67 dropped out before delivery. Among the 389 live born, singleton infants, our analysis included mother-child pairs that had at least one measure of child IQ at ages 5 or 8 years, at least one urinary phthalate concentration during gestation and childhood, and no missing covariate information (n=7). We further restricted the analytic sample to include only children who were Black or White. Our final sample included 253 mother-child pairs (see supplemental Figure S1).

Urinary phthalate metabolite concentration assessment

Study staff collected maternal urine samples at approximately 16-and 26-weeks gestation in polypropylene specimen cups. We collected child urine samples at ages 1, 2, 3, 4, 5, and 8 years. Among children who were not toilet trained, we collected urine by placing surgical inserts in clean diapers. We lined training potties with inserts to collect urine from children who were in the process of being toilet-trained. Urine from inserts was collected with a syringe and expressed into a collection cup in the laboratory. For children who were toilet-trained, caregivers assisted in the collection of urine using polypropylene specimen cups. We followed previously described protocols to minimize external contamination of urine samples (46, 47). All urine samples were refrigerated for less than 24 hours before processing, and stored at ≤ -20°C until chemical analysis at the Centers for Disease Control and Prevention (CDC).

Using a modified method of on-line solid phase extraction coupled with isotope dilution high performance liquid chromatography-tandem mass spectrometry, CDC staff measured the urinary phthalate metabolite concentrations (13). We measured urinary concentrations of mono(3-carboxypropyl) phthalate (MCPP), mono-isobutyl phthalate (MiBP), monobenzyl phthalate (MBzP), mono-n-butyl phthalate (MBP), monocarboxyoctyl phthalate (MCOP), monocarboxynonyl phthalate (MCNP) and monoethyl phthalate (MEP). We used three oxidative DEHP metabolites (mono-2-ethyl-5- hydroxyhexyl phthalate [MEHHP], mono-2-ethyl-5-oxohexyl phthalate [MEOHP], and mono-2-ethyl-5-carboxypentyl phthalate

[MECPP]) to create a summary DEHP metabolite measure (i.e., ΣDEHP) for both gestational and childhood samples. To calculate concentrations of ΣDEHP (in ng/mL), we divided each DEHP metabolite concentration by its molar mass, summed the individual concentrations, and then multiplied the molar sum by the molar mass of MECPP (48).

We did not measure MCOP or MCNP concentrations from maternal urine samples, because the method for these biomarkers had not yet been developed. We could not measure concentrations of MBP, MiBP, or MEHP from child urine samples collected at ages 1-3 years, as these metabolites were detected within the diaper inserts used during collection (9). The limits of detection (LODs) for the phthalate metabolites ranged from ~0.1 to ~1 ng/mL. Values below the LOD were given a value of the LOD/√2 (see supplemental Table S3) (49). To account for urine dilution, we measured urinary creatinine concentrations using previously described methods (50).

Phthalate metabolite concentrations (ng/mL) were creatinine-standardized, $\log_{10}$-transformed, and measurement-error corrected. Briefly, we accounted for phthalate exposure measurement error using a previously a described regression-calibration approach (51). For gestational phthalate concentrations, we used a random intercept linear mixed model to estimate geometric mean creatinine-standardized urinary phthalate concentrations across the two measurement occasions (i.e., 16 and 26 weeks) (52). While this calibration approach is appropriate when geometric mean phthalate concentrations show no time trends across measurement occasions, this was not the case for childhood concentrations, which varied quadratically with child age (47). Therefore, we used a more complex linear mixed effects model was used to account for measurement error in childhood phthalate measures.

To account for individual variation in urinary phthalate metabolite concentrations at multiple timepoints during childhood, we used linear mixed models to estimate the relation between age and $\log_{10}$-transformed creatinine-standardized phthalate metabolite concentrations as a function of age and age-squared from age 1-8 years. We included subject-specific intercepts and linear age slopes. For each subject, we used the estimated best linear unbiased predictor (eBLUP) to calculate phthalate metabolite concentrations at each time point and averaged across childhood. The average childhood value was calculated by dividing the area under the estimated trajectories of phthalate metabolite concentrations curve by the length of time (age 1-8 years). This method accounts for measurement error, individual variation in the number of samples ascertained, and exposure time trends in urinary phthalate metabolite concentrations.

For the rest of the manuscript, we refer to these measurement-error corrected values as urinary phthalate metabolite concentrations.

Cognitive outcomes

Children's cognitive abilities were assessed by three trained examiners using the Wechsler Preschool and Primary Scale of Intelligence-III (WPPSI-III) at age five years, and the Wechsler Intelligence Scale for Children-IV (WISC-IV) at age 8 years (53–55). Following initial training and certification on these assessments, quality control checks were unannounced, and completed (by KY) every six months to ensure IQ measures were properly administered and accurately scored. Both instruments assess children's overall intellectual abilities (Full-Scale Intelligence Quotient [FSIQ]) based on subscales for verbal comprehension, working memory, processing speed and others. In this analysis, we focused on FSIQ as our primary outcome of interest. The FSIQ scores from the WPPSI-III are comparable to those from the WISC-IV and thus we averaged them if more than one measurement was available (53, 54). We used standardized FSIQ scores (i.e., mean=100 and standard deviation (SD=15)) based on US normative data. Higher scores indicate better cognitive performance.

Covariate assessment

We used directed acyclic graphs (DAGs) to identify potential confounders that may be associated with both race and IQ, considering how confounders may bias the association between race and child IQ through exposure to phthalates during gestation and childhood (see supplemental Figure S2 and S3). Sociodemographic and maternal factors were collected using standardized questionnaires, administered by trained reviewers. Child sex was abstracted from hospital medical charts (56). We derived maternal pre-pregnancy body mass index (BMI) using self-reported height and weight, and imputed weight for mothers with missing data (57). We assessed secondhand and active tobacco smoke exposure during pregnancy by averaging cotinine concentrations from serum collected at 16- and 26-weeks gestation. Previously established thresholds to determine active, second-hand, and non-smoking (unexposed) using serum cotinine were ≥3.0 ng/mL, <3.0- ≥0.015 ng/mL, and

<0.015 ng/mL, respectively (58). Maternal cognitive abilities were assessed when children were ≥1 years using the, Wechsler Abbreviated Scale of Intelligence (59). In primary analyses, we adjusted for maternal age, pre-pregnancy BMI, household income, $\log_{10}$-transformed cotinine concentration, and maternal FSIQ scores.

Statistical analyses

First, we calculated univariate summary statistics and characterized distributions of study sample characteristics such as maternal sociodemographic and reproductive factors by child race. We further explored the distribution of urinary phthalate metabolite concentrations across visits by calculating univariate statistics and creating violin plots (60).

We calculated mean child 5 FSIQ scores by strata of the key covariates stratified by race. To maximize sample size and accommodate our modeling approach, we averaged repeated measures of FSIQ scores at ages 5 and 8 years when both were available. We assessed associations between average FSIQ scores with average phthalate concentrations during gestation and childhood, as well as average FSIQ scores with time-point specific phthalate concentrations. However, in cases where we examined phthalate concentrations at age 8 years, we used FSIQ collected only at age 8 years to ensure proper temporal ordering.

Mediation analyses

First, we quantified the racial disparities in child FSIQ scores. We used a linear regression model to estimate unadjusted and covariate-adjusted difference in FSIQ scores between Black and White children. This represents the total effect. Second, we examined racial disparities in average gestational and childhood urinary phthalate metabolite concentrations by examining univariate statistics and percent differences in concentrations of urinary phthalate metabolites between Black and White children.

Third, for phthalates that differed by race, we conducted mediation analyses following previously established methods for evaluating health disparities by Bellavia and colleagues (44). We evaluated if associations between child race and average FSIQ score were mediated by gestational or childhood urinary phthalate metabolite concentrations using the R package, Mediation (44, 61). This package estimates the average causal indirect effects, average direct effects, and total effects based previously established methods for linear structural equation modeling (62).

We estimated the covariate adjusted, average direct (association between race and child FSIQ), and average indirect effects (association between race and child FSIQ through average gestational and childhood urinary phthalate concentrations). Note that in models of average phthalate metabolite concentrations for childhood, we only included phthalate concentrations from ages 1, 2, 3, 4, and 5 years, as the outcome of childhood FSIQ score included values from age 5 and 8 years.

To assess mediation by average gestational and childhood urinary phthalate concentrations, we focused on the natural indirect effect, which is the effect of child race on FSIQ that operates only by changing the value of urinary phthalate metabolite concentrations, as this provides information on the pathways where disparities in child FSIQ originate. We also present the controlled direct effects, which is the effect of child race on child FSIQ score after fixing values of urinary phthalate concentrations (see supplemental Figure S4).

Secondary and Sensitivity Analyses

We conducted two secondary analyses. First, in cases where we identified racial differences in average child urinary phthalate metabolite concentrations, we further investigated if differences in urinary phthalate concentrations were also present at individual timepoints during childhood at ages 1,2,3,4,5 and 8 years. Second, for the same previously selected phthalate metabolites, we conducted mediation analyses to quantify the total, direct, and indirect effects of phthalate metabolites on the association between child race and average child FSIQ at individual time points during childhood. Note that for mediation analyses at age 8 years, child FSIQ at age 8 was used as the outcome (as opposed to average child FSIQ, which includes FSIQ scores ascertained at age 5 and 8 years).

We conducted several sensitivity analyses to assess the robustness of our results to various adjustments. In addition to previously specified covariates, we adjusted for child sex, quality and quantity of caregiving environment as measured using the Home Observation for Measurement of the Environment (HOME Inventory) (63), blood lead levels, and neighborhood socioeconomic position. HOME Inventory measures were assessed by study staff during home visits when children were age 1 year. The HOME Inventory is designed to measure the quality and quantity of stimulation and support available to children in their home, rather than socioeconomic position or quality of parenting (63). We collected whole blood samples from women at 16 and 26-weeks gestation and children at ages 1, 2, 3, 4, 5, and 8 years using collection materials prescreened for lead contamination (64). Blood lead concentrations were quantified at the Centers for Disease Control and Prevention laboratories using inductively coupled plasma mass spectrometry (65). Neighborhood socioeconomic position among HOME study participants was previously assessed using data from 2000 United States Census Records (68, 69). We conducted statistical analyses using R Studio (version 4.0.3; R Development Core Team) (70).

Breaking the cycle of children's environmental health disparities

The International Cycle of Environmental Health Disparities perpetuates through the intersectionality of many systems, identified in Figure 1 (71). This project will work towards breaking the cycle of children's environmental health disparities through four main avenues. First, this work identifies racial disparities in Health Outcomes by focusing on child cognitive abilities as the primary outcome of interest. Second, we aim to identify disparities in children's cognitive abilities based on differential exposure to environmental chemicals, focusing primarily on phthalates. Third, this work has the potential to influence social, cultural, and economic change through consumer education of phthalate containing products, so individuals can become aware of their exposure potential and impact and become informed in order to alter behavior patterns and reduce exposure. Finally, future implications for this work may challenge residential realities, which include societal level factors imposed on individuals within a given community. For example, findings from this work may be used to combat producer imposed white beauty standards and racially targeting marketing of personal care products containing phthalates and other harmful chemicals. Targeting multiple elements of the International Cycle of Environmental Health Disparities is necessary to dismantle environmental injustice, to ultimately break the cycle of children's environmental health disparities.

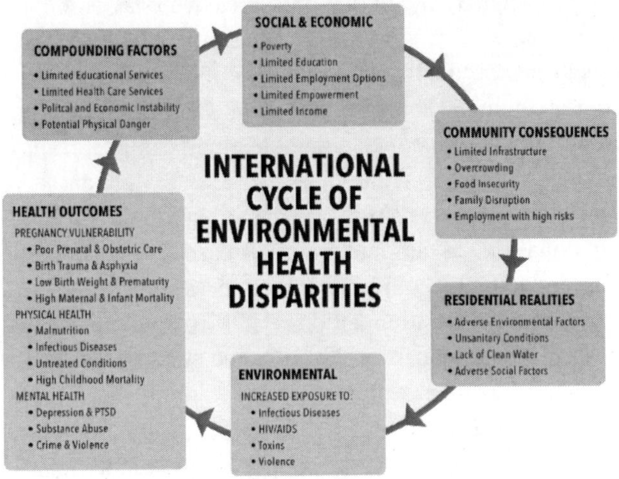

International Cycle of Environmental Health Disparities

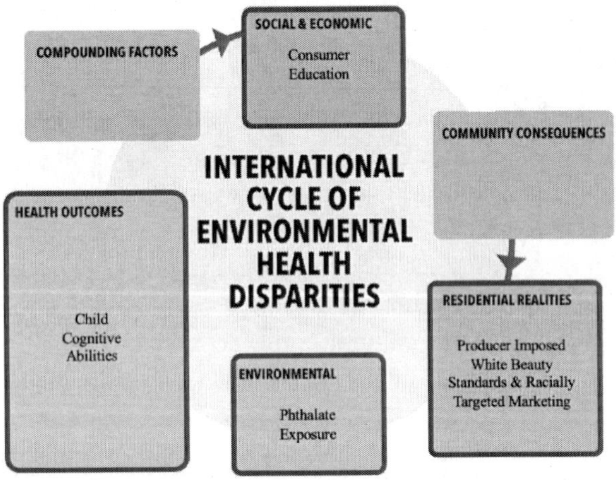

Breaking the Cycle of Environmental Health Disparities

Figure 1. Dismantling the International Cycle of Environmental Health Disparities by investigating racial disparities in children's cognitive abilities modified by early life phthalate exposure. This figure was adapted from previously published work (71). This work contributes to breaking the cycle of environmental health disparities though four avenues, Social & Economic, Residential Realities, Environmental, and Health Outcomes. Disrupting the International Cycle of Environmental Health Disparities in multiple ways will contribute to breaking the cycle and preventing it from continuing.

Our findings

Among 253 mother-child pairs, 38% (n=90) were Black children and 62% (n=145) were White children. Compared with White children, Black children were more likely to have mothers who were younger (<25 years at the time of gestation) and had acquired less education, with lower household incomes, and who were more likely to smoke during pregnancy, be multiparous, and have higher pre-pregnancy Body Mass Index (BMI) (see Table 1, supplemental Table S1). For both Black and White children, FSIQ scores were positively associated with maternal age, maternal education, and household income (see Table 2).

Table 1. Characteristics of mother-child dyads with follow-up at age 5 and/or 8 years by child race, according to covariates: The HOME Study (2003-2006)

Variable	Full Sample	Black	White
	N (%)	N (%)	N (%)
Overall	253 (100)	90 (36)	145 (57)
Maternal Age			
<25 years	57 (23)	45 (50)	8 (5)
25 - <35 years	154 (61)	40 (44)	104 (72)
35+ years	42 (17)	5 (6)	33 (23)
Maternal Education			
High School or less	62 (25)	51 (57)	7 (5)
Some College	71 (28)	31 (34)	37 (26)
Completed College	120 (47)	8 (9)	101 (70)
Maternal Race			
Non-Hispanic Black	83 (33)	82 (91)	1 (0)
Non-Hispanic White	152 (60)	5 (6)	142 (98)
Other	18 (7)	3 (3)	2 (1)
Annual Income			
<$30,000	82 (32)	70 (78)	9 (6)
$30,000 - $75,000	77 (30)	17 (19)	55 (38)
≥$75,000	94 (37)	3 (3)	81 (56)
Maternal Smoking [a]			
Unexposed	78 (31)	5 (6)	66 (56)
Second-Hand Smoking	116 (46)	40 (44)	71 (49)
Active Smoking	59 (23)	45 (50)	8 (6)
Parity			
0	114 (45)	29 (32)	73 (50)
1	79 (31)	29 (32)	46 (32)
2 +	60 (24)	32 (36)	26 (18)

Table 1. (Continued)

Variable	Full Sample N (%)	Black N (%)	White N (%)
Pre-pregnancy BMI (kg/m2)			
Normal/Underweight <25	125 (49)	32 (36)	83 (57)
Overweight ≥25 - <30	65 (26)	23 (26)	38 (26)
Obese ≥30	63 (25)	35 (39)	24 (17)
Child Sex			
Female	140 (55)	57 (63)	76 (52)

HOME Study: Health Outcomes and Measures of the Environment Stud, BMI: Body Mass Index.
[a] Maternal smoking during pregnancy estimated based on maternal serum cotinine concentrations during pregnancy. Unexposed smoking exposure defined as having serum cotinine concentrations <0.015ng/mL, second-hand smoking exposure is defined by serum cotinine concentrations between 0.015 and <3.00 ng/mL, and active smoking includes those with serum cotinine concentrations ≥ 3.00 ng/mL.
Note: percentages reflect columns (e.g., race) within each study sample characteristic.

Table 2. Full-scale intelligence quotient scores averaged [a] from ages 5 and 8 years according to covariates among mother-child dyads with child race, according to covariates: The HOME Study (2003-2006)

	Non-Hispanic Black		Non-Hispanic White	
Variable	N	Mean ± SD	N	Mean ± SD
Overall	90	91 ± 13	145	107 ± 12
Maternal Age				
<25 years	45	89 ± 15	8	101 ± 14
25 - <35 years	40	91 ± 11	104	107 ± 12
35+ years	5	103 ± 13	33	108 ± 13
Maternal Education				
High School or less	51	88 ± 14	7	98 ± 17
Some College	31	92 ± 13	37	103 ± 13
Completed College	8	102 ± 5.9	101	109 ± 11
Annual Income				
<$30,000	70	89 ± 14	9	98 ± 19
$30,000 - $75,000	17	95 ± 11	55	104 ± 12
≥$75,000	3	103 ± 6.6	81	110 ± 10
Maternal Smoking [b]				
Unexposed	5	96 ± 7.2	66	106 ± 12
Second-Hand Smoking	40	91 ± 12	71	107 ± 13
Active Smoking	45	91 ± 17	8	111 ± 17
Parity				
0	29	88 ± 14	73	109 ± 13
1	29	91 ± 13	46	107 ± 10
2 +	32	93 ± 13	26	103 ± 12
Pre-pregnancy BMI (kg/m2)				
Normal/Underweight <25	32	88 ± 15	83	108 ± 12

	Non-Hispanic Black		Non-Hispanic White	
Variable	**N**	**Mean ± SD**	**N**	**Mean ± SD**
Overweight ≥25 - <30	23	95 ± 11	38	107 ± 13
Obese ≥30	35	90 ± 13	24	104 ± 14
Child Sex				
Male	33	89 ± 13	69	105 ± 13
Female	57	92 ± 14	76	109 ± 12

HOME Study: Health Outcomes and Measures of the Environment Study, BMI: Body Mass Index, FSIQ: Full Scale Intelligence Quotient

[a] Average FSIQ values represent the arithmetic mean of repeated child FSIQ Scores. In cases where children only had one FSIQ measure, that value was used to represent the mean. Of the full analytic sample (n=253), n=169 children had two measures of FSIQ ascertained at 5 and 8 years (67%)

[b] Maternal smoking during pregnancy estimated based on maternal serum cotinine concentrations during pregnancy. Unexposed smoking exposure defined as having serum cotinine concentrations <0.015ng/mL, second-hand smoking exposure is defined by serum cotinine concentrations between 0.015 and <3.00 ng/mL, and active smoking includes those with serum cotinine concentrations ≥3.00 ng/mL.

Table 3. Unadjusted and adjusted [a] difference in child FSIQ at age 5 and/or 8 years by child race: The HOME Study (2003-2006)

FSIQ Measure		Difference Black vs. White (95% CI) [b]			
	N	Unadjusted		Adjusted	
5 Year FSIQ	187	-17.0	(-21.0, -13.1)	-7.6	(-13.5, -1.7)
8 Year FSIQ	207	-17.4	(-21.2, -13.7)	-9.6	(-15.5, -3.7)
Average FSIQ [c]	235	-16.0	(-19.4, -12.7)	-7.0	(-12.1, -1.8)

FSIQ: Full Scale Intelligence Quotient, HOME Study: Health Outcomes and Measures of the Environment Study.

[a] Adjusted for maternal age (continuous), pre-pregnancy BMI (continuous), income (continuous), log-10 transformed average gestational cotinine concentration (continuous), and maternal FSIQ scores (continuous).

[b] Values depict the difference in FSIQ scores between Black and White children, where White children are the reference group.

[c] Average FSIQ values represent the arithmetic mean of repeated child FSIQ Scores. In cases where children only had one FSIQ measure, that value was used to represent the mean.

In unadjusted analyses, FSIQ scores among Black children were 16 points lower (β: -16.0 95% CI: -19.4, -12.7) compared with White Children (see Table 3). After adjusting for covariates, Black children had FSIQ scores 7-points (β: -7.0 95% CI -12.1, -1.8) lower than White children after adjusting for covariates.

Univariate statistics: Mediators (phthalate metabolites)

Urinary MCPP, MiBP, MBzP, MBP, and ΣDEHP concentrations were lower during gestation relative to childhood (see Figure 2, supplemental Table S2 and S3). During gestation and childhood, MBzP (gestation percent difference: 16, 95% CI: 13, 21; childhood percent difference: 13, 95% CI: 12, 15) and MEP (gestation percent difference: 15, 95% CI: 11, 19; childhood percent difference: 21, 95% CI: 19, 24) concentrations were higher in Black children compared with White Children (see Figure 3, supplemental Table S2 and S3). During pregnancy, urinary ΣDEHP concentrations were higher in White mothers than Black mothers. All other phthalate metabolite concentrations were similar during gestation and childhood in Black and White participants (percent differences for average gestation or average childhood <13.0) (see Figure 2). Thus, for subsequent analyses, we focused on MBzP and MEP concentrations.

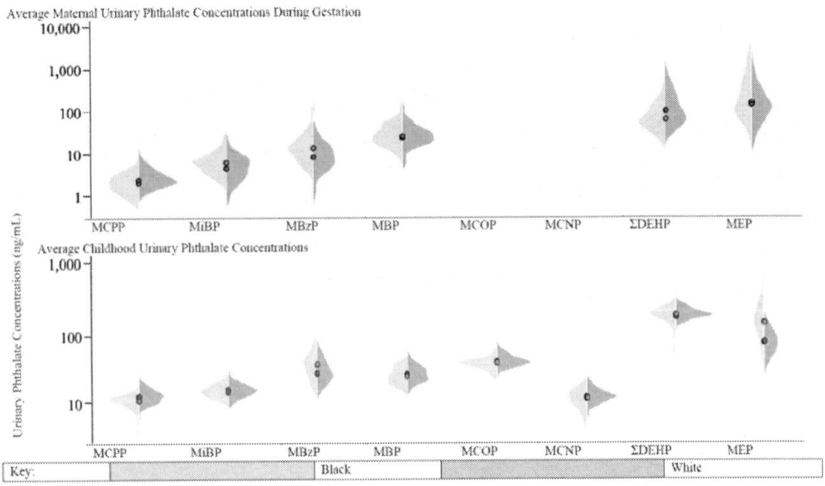

Figure 2. Violin plots of error corrected urinary phthalate metabolite concentrations averaged for gestation and childhood periods among mother-child dyads: The HOME Study (2003-2006). HOME Study (Health and Measures of the Environment Study); MCPP, mono(3- carboxypropyl) phthalate; MiBP, mono-isobutyl phthalate; MBzP, monobenzyl phthalate; MBP, mono-n-butyl phthalate; MCOP, monocarboxyoctyl phthalate; MCNP, monocarboxynonyl phthalate; ΣDEHP, summary di(2-ethylhexyl) phthalate metabolite measure; MEP, monoethyl phthalate The shaded area represents the density function of phthalate metabolite concentrations, and the dot represents the median. Repeated maternal urinary phthalate metabolites assessed at 16 and 26 weeks gestation.

Repeated child urinary phthalate metabolites assessed at age 1, 2, 3, 4, and 5 years. Note, the average value of urinary phthalate concentrations does not include those collected at age 8 year since the primary outcome, average FSIQ consists of scores from age 5 and 8 years. Concentrations of ΣDEHP (in ng/mL) were calculated using the following formula: ΣDEHP (ng/mL)=[MECPP (ng/mL)/308.33 g/mol + MEHHP (ng/mL)/294.347 g/mol + MEOHP (ng/mL)/292.331 g/mol] * 308.33 g/mol.

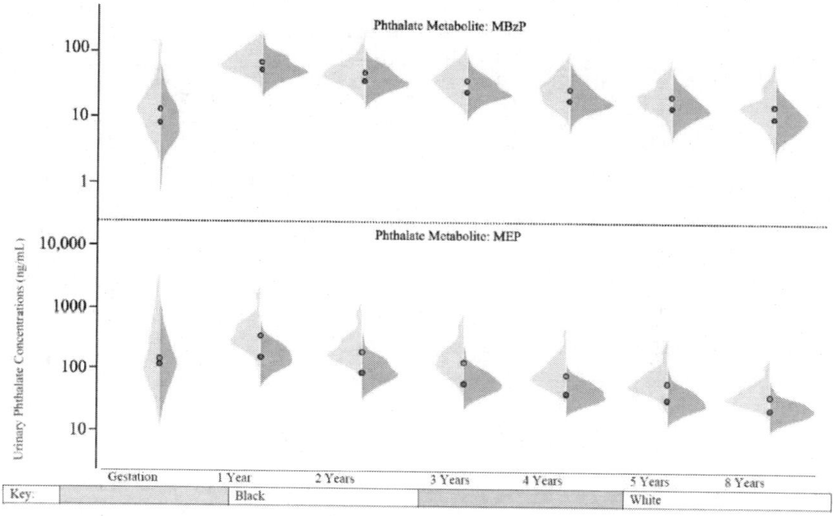

Figure 3. Violin plots of error corrected urinary phthalate metabolite concentrations during gestation and childhood among mother-child dyads: The HOME Study (2003-2006). HOME Study (Health and Measures of the Environment Study); MBzP, monobenzyl phthalate; MEP: monoethyl phthalate. The shaded area represents the density function of phthalate metabolite concentrations, and the dot represents the median. Repeated maternal urinary phthalate metabolites assessed at 16 and 26 weeks gestation.

Mediation analyses

Gestational phthalate metabolite concentrations did not contribute to racial disparities in child FSIQ (see Table 4). Average childhood MEP concentrations showed modest evidence for mediation. The natural indirect effect of 10-fold increase in average childhood MEP concentrations contributed to -1.1 point (95% CI: -3.0, 0.8) difference in the Black-White FSIQ disparity, though the confidence interval includes the null. The direct effect of race on child FSIQ scores, controlling for average childhood MEP concentration, modestly decreased (β: -5.8 95% CI: -12, -0.4).

Table 4. Adjusted [a] direct and indirect associations between child race and average child FSIQ scores at ages 5 and/or 8 years [b], mediated through gestational and childhood error corrected urinary phthalate metabolite concentrations [b]: The HOME Study (2003-2006)

Metabolite	Visit	Gestation [c]		P-value	Childhood [d]		P-value
		β (95% CI)		P-value	*β* (95% CI)		P-value
MCPP	Direct Effect	-6.7	(-11.9, -1.6)	0.01	-8.6	(-13.8, -3.3)	<0.01
	Indirect Effect	-0.2	(-1.7, 1.3)	0.82	1.5	(0.2, 3.2)	0.02
MiBP	Direct Effect	-7.0	(-12.3, 1.9)	<0.01	-7.1	(-12.2, -1.9)	0.01
	Indirect Effect	0.1	(-0.3, 0.7)	0.72	0.0	(-0.7, 0.5)	0.86
MBzP	Direct Effect	-7.2	(-12.6, -1.5)	0.02	-7.4	(-12.2, -2.3)	<0.01
	Indirect Effect	0.1	(-0.4, 0.7)	0.77	0.5	(-0.3, 1.7)	0.23
MBP	Direct Effect	-7.0	(-11.5, -1.9)	<0.01	-6.9	(-11.9, -1.9)	<0.01
	Indirect Effect	-0.1	(-0.5, 0.3)	0.81	-0.1	(-0.9, 0.5)	0.70
MCNP [e]	Direct Effect	--	--	--	-7.1	(-12.5, -1.7)	0.01
	Indirect Effect	--	--	--	0.0	(-0.7, 0.7)	0.91
MCOP [e]	Direct Effect	--	--	--	-7.1	(-12.2, -1.6)	<0.01
	Indirect Effect	--	--	--	0.1	(-0.6, 1.0)	0.72
ΣDEHP [f]	Direct Effect	-6.3	(-11.8, -1.0)	0.01	-7.0	(-12.3, -1.7)	0.01
	Indirect Effect	-0.6	(-1.9, 0.4)	0.21	0.0	(-0.7, 0.7)	0.92
MEP	Direct Effect	-7.0	(-12.2, -2.0)	<0.01	-5.8	(-11.6, -0.4)	0.03
	Indirect Effect	0.1	(-0.4, 0.8)	0.78	-1.1	(-3.0, 0.8)	0.24

FSIQ: Full Scale Intelligence Quotient, HOME Study: Health Outcomes and Measures of the Environment Study

MCPP, mono(3- carboxypropyl) phthalate; MiBP, mono-isobutyl phthalate; MBzP, monobenzyl phthalate; MBP, mono-n-butyl phthalate; MCOP, monocarboxyoctyl phthalate; MCNP, monocarboxynonyl phthalate; ΣDEHP, summary di(2-ethylhexyl) phthalate metabolite measure; MEP, monoethyl phthalate

[a] Adjusted for maternal age (continuous), pre-pregnancy BMI (continuous), income (continuous), log-10 transformed average gestational cotinine concentration (continuous), and maternal FSIQ scores (continuous)

[b] Average FSIQ values represent the arithmetic mean of repeated child FSIQ Scores. In cases where children only had one FSIQ measure, that value was used to represent the mean.

[c] Repeated maternal urinary phthalate metabolites assessed at 16 and 26 weeks gestation

[d] Repeated child urinary phthalate metabolites assessed at age 1, 2, 3, 4, and 5 years. Note, the average value of urinary phthalate concentrations does not include those collected at age 8 year since the primary outcome, average FSIQ consists of scores from age 5 and 8 years.

[e] We did not measure MCNP or MCOP concentrations from maternal urine samples, as the method for these biomarkers had not yet been developed at the time of analysis

[f] Concentrations of ΣDEHP (in ng/mL) were calculated using the following formula: ΣDEHP (ng/mL)=[MECPP (ng/mL)/308.33 g/mol + MEHHP (ng/mL)/294.347 g/mol + MEOHP (ng/mL)/292.331 g/mol] * 308.33 g/mol

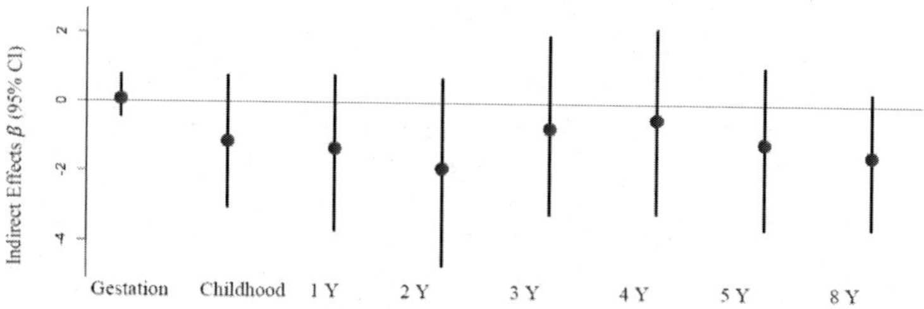

Figure 4. Adjusted indirect associations between child race and average child FSIQ at ages 5 and/or 8 years mediated through gestational and childhood urinary MEP concentrations: The HOME Study (2003-2006). FSIQ: Full Scale Intelligence Quotient; HOME: Health Outcomes and Measures of the Environment Study; MEP, monoethyl phthalate. Adjusted for maternal age (continuous), pre-pregnancy BMI (continuous), income (continuous), log-10 transformed average gestational cotinine concentration (continuous), and maternal FSIQ scores (continuous). Repeated maternal urinary phthalate metabolites assessed at 16 and 26 weeks gestation. Repeated child urinary phthalate metabolites assessed at age 1, 2, 3, 4, and 5 years. Note, the average value of urinary phthalate concentrations does not include those collected at age 8 year since the primary outcome, average FSIQ consists of scores from age 5 and 8 years.

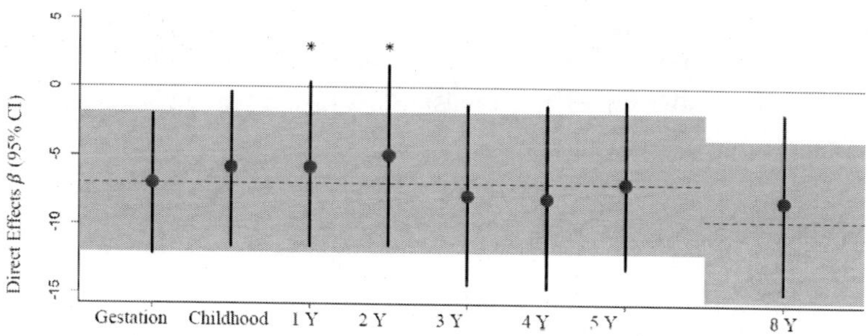

Figure 5. Adjusted direct associations between child race and average child FSIQ at ages 5 or 8 years before (dotted line and gray band) and after (point and whisker) controlling for gestational or childhood urinary MEP concentrations: The HOME Study (2003-2006). FSIQ: Full Scale Intelligence Quotient; HOME: Health Outcomes and Measures of the Environment Study; MEP, monoethyl phthalate. Adjusted for maternal age (continuous), pre-pregnancy BMI (continuous), income (continuous), log-10 transformed average gestational cotinine concentration (continuous), and maternal FSIQ scores (continuous). Repeated maternal urinary phthalate metabolites assessed at 16- and 26-weeks gestation. Repeated child urinary phthalate metabolites assessed at age 1, 2, 3, 4, and 5 years. Note, the average value of urinary phthalate concentrations does not include those collected at age 8 year since the primary outcome, average FSIQ consists of scores from age 5 and 8 years.

The shaded area and dashed line represents the total effect of child race on average child FSIQ score. Note that the total effect for average FSIQ score only corresponds to timepoints assessed prior to age 8 years. The total effect for age 8 years is specific to the FSIQ score obtained at age 8 years. The solid horizontal line at 0 indicates no difference in racial disparities in child FSIQ scores. The asterisk indicates a non-significant controlled direct effect.

The natural indirect effects of MEP on IQ appeared to be stronger during early childhood (see Figure 3). The strongest natural indirect effect of MEP on child FSIQ scores was observed at age two years (β = -1.9, 95% CI: -4.7, 0.7) (see supplemental Table S4). While the 95% CI of the indirect effect estimate included the null value, the residual disparity, or adjusted direct associations in FSIQ after controlling for MEP, was attenuated to less than 5 points (β = -4.9, 95% CI: -11.5, 1.6) (see Figure 5).

Sensitivity analyses

We conducted sensitivity analyses for phthalate metabolite MEP. In addition to previously identified covariates, adjusting for child sex or caregiving environment (HOME scores) did not substantially change the pattern of results (supplemental Table S5). Additional adjustment for maternal neighborhood socioeconomic position during gestation reduced the racial disparity in child FSIQ scores from 7.0 points (95% CI: -12.1, -1.8) to 6.1 points (95% CI: -11.7, -0.6). Adjusting for time-point specific blood lead levels during gestation and childhood also resulted in decreasing in the disparity in child FSIQ scores, particularly in early childhood.

Discussion

By applying mediation methods to a longitudinal birth cohort, we sought to determine if racial disparities in children's cognitive abilities could be explained, in part, by higher early life exposure to phthalates. During gestation and early childhood, urinary concentrations of MBzP and MEP were higher among Black children than White children. Furthermore, average child FSIQ scores were 7-points lower among Black children than White children after adjusting for socioeconomic factors. We did not observe compelling evidence that phthalate concentrations mediated racial disparities in child FSIQ. Only childhood urinary MEP concentrations modestly mediated racial disparities in IQ scores.

Overall, we found that only MEP weakly mediated the association between race and child FSIQ. We are unaware of any studies evaluating the role of phthalates in mediating this association. Other investigators have documented racial disparities in child FSIQ, (31–33) and differences in phthalate exposure across racial groups (13, 38–40, 43). Moreover, some studies report associations between gestational and early life phthalate exposure with decreased child IQ (16–22, 24, 25). Direct and indirect effects of all phthalate metabolites showed an inverse association with child cognitive abilities, with the exception of MCPP during childhood (β: 1.5 points; 95% CI: 0.2, 3.2). This finding was counterintuitive, as we did not expect phthalates to have a protective effect; however, these results could be spurious as most indirect coefficients were centered around the null. Further, MCPP is a non-specific phthalate metabolite, as it represents a breakdown product of several other higher molecular weight phthalate diesters.[70] Urinary concentrations of MCPP were also the lowest of all phthalate metabolites assessed, which could also contribute to these findings. Consistent with our prior work using the HOME Study, higher urinary MEP concentrations during childhood were associated with lower FSIQ (16). The lack of stronger mediating effects might be due to the relatively modest association that MEP and other phthalates have with child cognitive abilities. Further, given that adjustment for socioeconomic and environmental factors attenuated the racial differences in IQ by almost half of a standard deviation in IQ scores, additional environmental factors are likely to play a major role in explaining racial disparities in IQ. This is further evidenced by the multiple factors identified by the International Cycle of Environmental Health Disparities, which identifies how health disparities perpetuate through the combined impacts of multiple risk factors both the individual and societal level.

MEP is of particular interest for several reasons. First, urinary concentrations of MEP are substantially higher in Black populations than White (5, 71, 72). Independent of socioeconomic position, Black women have higher body burdens of some phthalates, and other environmental chemical exposures than White women, partly due to consumer beauty product use (38, 73–75). Second, diethyl phthalate (DEP), the parent compound of MEP, is commonly used in a variety of consumer products such as make-up, nail polish, perfume, deodorant, and various hair products (spray, dyes, mousse, crème rinse, nutrients, and conditioners) (5, 25–28, 71, 76). Thus, MEP may represent a marker for multiple compounds used within these products, which could induce co-pollutant confounding. The primary route of exposure for DEP is dermal absorption and suggests that frequent use of DEP containing products may result in higher internal body burdens of MEP compared to phthalates with different routes of exposure (71). Some of these products are heavily marketed to Black communities, highlighting how cosmetics can be an environmental injustice (77). Differences in exposure to phthalate containing products could in part be due to discriminative advertising practices, (78, 79) directed to maintain European, White beauty standards (i.e., hair relaxers and skin lighteners) (80, 81).

Our study has some limitations. First, the sample size was modest, and it varied during follow up, from gestation through childhood; we retained fewer Black families than White families, which may result in selection bias. The reductions in sample size due to loss to follow-up also reduce statistical power, limiting our ability to observe subtler associations. Second, measures of child cognition, including assessing IQ, are historically controversial (26–30). Despite efforts to reduce racial, ethic, and socioeconomic biases in tools for assessing intelligence, some biases remain (31, 33, 37). Third, we were unable to consider multiple mediators in our analysis to consider both sources of phthalate exposure (i.e., daily personal care product use, fast food consumption) in addition to phthalate biomarkers, as recommended by Bellavia et al. (44). While assessing urinary concentrations of phthalate metabolites can provide an assessment of phthalate exposure from multiple sources, it remains difficult to directly translate these findings to personal recommendations or policy (44). For example it may be more practical to intervene on behavior patterns related to phthalate containing product use as a modifiable exposure, rather than any one specific phthalate metabolite (1). Future work could consider phthalate exposure sources, such as hair or beauty products, in addition to biomarkers of phthalates when investigating racial disparities in child FSIQ. Fourth, while we adjusted for many relevant covariates, residual confounding remains a possibility. For example, adjusting for income as a measure of socioeconomic status may not fully capture the cumulative effects of daily experiences for minority populations, such as racism, chronic psychosocial stress, inequitable education opportunities, and other environmental exposures (33, 37). Further, given that adjustment for socioeconomic and environmental factors attenuated the racial differences in IQ by almost half of a standard deviation in IQ scores, additional environmental factors are likely to play a major role in explaining racial disparities in IQ. It is also important to recognize that race is a social construct, rather than a biological variable. As such, including race as a variable in our models does not capture the totality of minority and marginalized peoples' experience that impact child cognitive development.

This study had several strengths. First, we had extensive biomarkers of phthalate exposure from the 2nd trimester of pregnancy until children were age 8 years, along with up to two measures of cognitive ability. This is a notable because most published studies only had one phthalate biomarker, which is subject to substantial within-person variation due to the episodic nature of phthalate exposure and the short half-life of phthalates (3, 9, 82, 83). Second, we used regression calibration to repeated urinary phthalate concentrations from gestation and early childhood to account for measurement error. Third, we applied advanced epidemiological methods to evaluate phthalates as a source of racial disparities in child FSIQ (44).

Our findings have potential implications for future research and policies, particularly surrounding the use of phthalates in personal care and consumer products. We found that Black mothers and their children had higher exposure to several phthalate metabolites than Whites mothers and their children, probably personal care products marketed towards the Black community. Black women historically have been encouraged to alter their hair texture and styles to reflect White beauty standards, (77, 84–87) that may increase their exposure to toxic chemicals found in products such as hair relaxers. Additionally, companies producing such products advertise almost exclusively to the Black community, and consumers generally are often unaware of harmful chemical exposures (77–80, 88).

As scientific evidence of the harmful health effects of phthalates grows, phthalates and other harmful chemicals have been removed from some products, though these products tend to be more expensive and are generally marketed towards Whites (77). While behavior-based interventions to educate and empower consumers to make informed decisions of their personal care product use can reduce phthalate exposure,(89) eliminating phthalates in consumer products is essential to eliminate exposure. Additionally, other exposures that have racial disparities should also be considered in this context (e.g., PBDEs and IQ) (90).

Conclusion

We observed racial disparities in child cognition and exposure to some phthalates during gestation, infancy, and childhood. Overall, we did not observe compelling evidence that phthalates mediated racial disparities in child IQ. However, children's urinary concentrations of MEP explained some, but not all, of the association between race and child IQ. Though we did not find overwhelming evidence for phthalates to mediate the association between race and child IQ, efforts to reduce exposure to known and suspected neurotoxicants, may diminish some of the disparities in cognitive abilities observed between Black and White children.

Acknowledgments

JMB served as an expert witness in litigation related to perfluorooctanonic acid contamination in drinking water in New Hampshire. Any funds he received from this arrangement were/are paid to Brown University and cannot be used for his direct benefit (e.g., salary/fringe, travel, etc). The results reported herein correspond to specific aims of grant R01 ES024381 to investigator Joseph M Braun, R01 ES020349 to investigators Aimin Chen, Bruce P Lanphear, and Kimberly Yolton, R01 ES011261 to investigator Bruce P. Lanphear, R01 ES014575 to investigators Bruce P. Lanphear and Kimberly Yolton from the National Institutes of Health. Computing code can be obtained from the corresponding author (MAP) upon request. Data from the HOME Study is available upon request. The HOME Study principal investigators have actively engaged in collaborative data-sharing projects. We welcome new collaborations with other investigators. Interested investigators in HOME Study data can explore data options at the following location: https://homestudy.research.cchmc.org/ and use the available link to contact the investigators to discuss collaborative opportunities. The Data Sharing Committee meets regularly to review proposed research projects and ensure that they do not overlap with extant projects and are an efficient use of scare resources (e.g., cord blood).

References

[1] Braun JM, Just AC, Williams PL, Smith KW, Calafat AM, Hauser R. Personal care product use and urinary phthalate metabolite and paraben concentrations during pregnancy among women from a fertility clinic. J Expo Sci Environ Epidemiol 2014;24:459–66. doi:10.1038/jes.2013.69.

[2] Carlstedt F, Jönsson BG, Bornehag CG. PVC flooring is related to human uptake of phthalates in infants. Indoor Air 2013;23:32–39. https://doi.org/10.1111/j.1600-0668.2012.00788.x.

[3] Hauser R, Calafat AM. Phthalates and human health. Occup Environ Med 2005;62:806–18. doi:10.1136/oem.2004.017590.

[4] Rudel RA, Gray JM, Engel CL, Rawsthorne TW, Dodson RE, Ackerman JM, Rizzo J, Nudelman JL, Brody JG. Food packaging and Bisphenol A and Bis(2-Ethyhexyl) phthalate exposure: Findings from a dietary intervention. Environ Health Perspect 2011;119:914–20. doi: 10.1289/ehp.1003170.

[5] Parlett LE, Calafat AM, Swan SH. Women's exposure to phthalates in relation to use of personal care products. J Expo Sci Environ Epidemiol 2013;23:197–206. doi:10.1038/jes.2012.105.

[6] Hernández-Díaz S, Su YC, Mitchell AA, Kelley KE, Calafat AM, Hauser R. Medications as a potential source of exposure to phthalates among women of childbearing age. Reprod Toxicol Elmsford N 2013;37:1–5. doi:10.1016/j.reprotox.2013.01.001.

[7] Agency for Toxic Substances and Disease Registry (ATSDR). Toxicological profile for Di(2-Ethylhexyl)phthalate (DEHP). Atlanta GA: Agency Toxic Subst Dis Regist, 2004.

[8] Bornehag CG, Lundgren B, Weschler CJ, Sigsgaard T, Hagerhed-Engman L, Sundell J. Phthalates in indoor dust and their association with building characteristics. Environ Health Perspect 2005;113:1399–404. doi:10.1289/ehp.7809.

[9] Watkins DJ, Eliot M, Sathyanarayana S, Calafat AM, Yolton K, Lanphear BP, Braun JM. Variability and predictors of urinary concentrations of phthalate metabolites during early childhood. Environ Sci Technol 2014;48:8881–90. doi:10.1021/es501744v.

[10] Woodruff TJ, Zota AR, Schwartz JM. Environmental chemicals in pregnant women in the United States: NHANES 2003-2004. Environ Health Perspect 2011;119:878–85. doi:10.1289/ehp.1002727.

[11] Koch HM, Preuss R, Drexler H, Angerer J. Exposure of nursery school children and their parents and teachers to Di-n-Butylphthalate and Butylbenzylphthalate. Int Arch Occup Environ Health 2005;78:223–9. doi:10.1007/s00420-004-0570-x.

[12] Koch HM, Drexler H, Angerer J. Internal exposure of nursery-school children and their parents and teachers to Di(2-Ethylhexyl)Phthalate (DEHP). Int J Hyg Environ Health 2004;207:15–22. doi: 10.1078/1438-4639-00270.

[13] Silva MJ, Barr DB, Reidy JA, Malek NA, Hodge CC, Caudill SP, Brock JW, Needham LL, Calafat AM. Urinary levels of seven phthalate metabolites in the US population from the National Health and Nutrition Examination Survey (NHANES) 1999-2000. Environ Health Perspect 2004;112:331–8. doi: 10.1289/ehp.6723.

[14] Sørensen LK. Determination of phthalates in milk and milk products by liquid chromatography/tandem mass spectrometry. Rapid Commun Mass Spectrom RCM 2006;20:1135–43. doi:10.1002/rcm.2425.

[15] Desvergne B, Feige JN. Casals-Casas, C. PPAR-mediated activity of phthalates: A link to the obesity epidemic? Mol Cell Endocrinol 2009;304:43–8. doi:10.1016/j.mce.2009.02.017.

[16] Li N, Papandonatos GD, Calafat AM, Yolton K, Lanphear BP, Chen A, Braun JM. Identifying periods of susceptibility to the impact of phthalates on children's cognitive abilities. Environ Res 2019;172:604–14. doi:10.1016/j.envres.2019.03.009.

[17] Doherty BT, Engel SM, Buckley JP, Silva MJ, Calafat AM, Wolff MS. Prenatal phthalate biomarker concentrations and performance on the Bayley Scales of Infant Development-II in a population of young urban children. Environ Res 2017;152:51–8. doi:10.1016/j.envres.2016.09.021.

[18] Factor-Litvak P, Insel B, Calafat AM, Liu X, Perera F, Rauh VA, Whyatt RM. Persistent associations between maternal prenatal exposure to phthalates on child IQ at age 7 years. PloS One 2014;9:e114003. doi:10.1371/journal.pone.0114003.

[19] Huang HB, Chen HY, Su PH, Huang PC, Sun CW, Wang CJ, Chen HY, Hsiung CA, Wang SL. Fetal and childhood exposure to phthalate diesters and cognitive function in children up to 12 years of age: Taiwanese maternal and infant cohort study. PloS One 2015;10:e0131910. doi:10.1371/journal.pone.0131910.

[20] Kim JI, Hong YC, Shin CH, Lee YA, Lim YH, Kim BN. The effects of maternal and children phthalate exposure on the neurocognitive function of 6-year-old children. Environ Res 2017;156:519–25. doi:10.1016/j.envres.2017.04.003.

[21] Kim S, Eom S, Kim HJ, Lee JJ, Choi G, Choi S, Kim S, Kim SY, Cho G, Kim YD, et al. Association between maternal exposure to major phthalates, heavy metals, and persistent organic pollutants, and the neurodevelopmental performances of their children at 1 to 2 years of age- CHECK Cohort Study. Sci Total Environ 2018;624:377–84. doi:10.1016/j.scitotenv.2017.12.058.

[22] Polanska K, Ligocka D, Sobala W, Hanke W. Phthalate exposure and child development: The Polish Mother and Child Cohort Study. Early Hum Dev 2014;90:477–85. doi:10.1016/j.earlhumdev.2014.06.006.

[23] Engel SM, Patisaul HB, Brody C, Hauser R, Zota AR, Bennet DH, Swanson M, Whyatt RM. Neurotoxicity of ortho-phthalates: Recommendations for critical policy reforms to protect brain development in children. Am J Public Health 2021;111:687–95. doi:10.2105/AJPH.2020.306014.

[24] Ipapo KN, Factor-Litvak P, Whyatt RM, Calafat AM, Diaz D, Perera F, Rauh V, Herbstman JB. Maternal prenatal urinary phthalate metabolite concentrations and visual recognition memory among infants at 27 weeks. Environ Res 2017;155:7–14. doi:10.1016/j.envres.2017.01.019.

[25] Téllez-Rojo MM, Cantoral A, Cantonwine DE, Schnaas L, Peterson K, Hu H, Meeker JD. Prenatal urinary phthalate metabolites levels and neurodevelopment in children at two and three years of age. Sci Total Environ 2013 Jun 05. doi:10.1016/j.scitotenv.2013.05.021.

[26] Gottfredson LS. Social consequences of group differences in cognitive ability. University of Delaware: Newark, DE, 2004. URL: http://www.udel.edu/educ/gottfredson/reprints/2004socialconsequences.pdf.

[27] Herrnstein RJ, Murray C. The bell curve: Intelligence and class structure in American life. New York: Free Press, 1994.

[28] Coyle TR, Pillow DR. SAT and ACT predict college GPA after removing g. intelligence 2008;36: 719–29. doi:10.1016/j.intell.2008.05.001.

[29] Schmidt FL, Hunter JE. The validity and utility of selection methods in personnel psychology: Practical and theoretical implications of 85 years of research findings. Psychol Bull 1998;124: 262–74. doi:10.1037/0033-2909.124.2.262.

[30] Schmidt FL, Hunter J. General mental ability in the world of work: Occupational attainment and job performance. J Pers Soc Psychol 2004;86:162–73. doi:10.1037/0022-3514.86.1.162.

[31] Thomas D. Racial IQ differences among transracial adoptees: fact or artifact? J Intell 2017;5:1. doi:10.3390/jintelligence5010001.

[32] Templer DI, Arikawa H. Association of race and color with mean IQ across nations. Psychol Rep 2006;99:191–6. doi:10.2466/pr0.99.1.191-196.

[33] LeWinn KZ, Bush NR, Batra A, Tylavsky F, Rehkopf D. Identification of modifiable social and behavioral factors associated with childhood cognitive performance. JAMA Pediatr 2020;174(11):1063-72. doi:10.1001/jamapediatrics.2020.2904.

[34] Rushton JP, Jensen AR. Thirty years of research on race differences in cognitive ability. Psychol Public Policy Law 2005;11:235–94. doi:10.1037/1076-8971.11.2.235.

[35] Lynn R. Race differences in intelligence: An evolutionary analysis. Augusta, GA: Washington Summit Books, 2006.

[36] Nisbett RE, Aronson J, Blair C, Dickens W, Flynn J, Halpern DF, Turkheimer E. Intelligence: New findings and theoretical developments. Am Psychol 2012;67:130–59. doi:10.1037/a0026699.

[37] Breslau N, Chilcoat HD, Susser ES, Matte T, Liang KY, Peterson EL. Stability and change in children's intelligence quotient scores: A comparison of two socioeconomically disparate communities. Am J Epidemiol 2001;154:711–17. doi:10.1093/aje/154.8.711.

[38] Kobrosly RW, Evans S, Miodovnik A, Barrett ES, Thurston SW, Calafat AM, Swan SH. Prenatal phthalate exposures and neurobehavioral development scores in boys and girls at 6-10 years of age. Environ Health Perspect 2014;122:521–8. doi:10.1289/ehp.1307063.

[39] James-Todd T, Meeker J, Huang T, Hauser R, Seely E, Ferguson K, Rich-Edwards J, McElrath T. Racial and ethnic variations in phthalate metabolite concentrations across pregnancy. J Expo Sci Environ Epidemiol 2017;27:160–6. doi:10.1038/jes.2016.2.

[40] Potischman N, Troisi R, Thadhani R, Hoover RN, Dodd K, Davis WW, Sluss PM, Hsieh CC, Ballard-Barbash R. Pregnancy hormone concentrations across ethnic groups: Implications for later cancer risk. Cancer Epidemiol Biomark Prev Publ Am Assoc Cancer Res Cosponsored Am Soc Prev Oncol 2005;14:1514–20. doi:10.1158/1055-9965.EPI-04-0869.

[41] Faupel-Badger JM, Wang Y, Karumanchi SA, Stanczyk F, Pollak M, McElrath T, Hoover RN, Troisi R. Associations of pregnancy characteristics with maternal and cord steroid hormones, angiogenic factors, and insulin-like growth factor Axis. Cancer Causes Control CCC 2011;22:1587–95. doi:10.1007/s10552-011-9835-3.

[42] Henderson BE, Bernstein L, Ross RK, Depue RH, Judd HL. The early in utero oestrogen and testosterone environment of Blacks and whites: Potential effects on male offspring. Br J Cancer 1988;57:216–8. doi:10.1038/bjc.1988.46.

[43] Huang T, Saxena AR, Isganaitis E, James-Todd T. Gender and racial/ethnic differences in the associations of urinary phthalate metabolites with markers of diabetes risk: National Health and Nutrition Examination Survey 2001–2008. Environ. Health 2014;13:6. doi:10.1186/1476-069X-13-6.

[44] Bellavia A, Zota AR, Valeri L, James-Todd T. Multiple mediators approach to study environmental chemicals as determinants of health disparities. Environ Epidemiol 2018;2(2):e015. doi:10.1097/EE9.0000000000000015.

[45] Braun JM, Kalloo G, Chen A, Dietrich KN, Liddy-Hicks S, Morgan S, Xu Y, Yolton K, Lanphear BP. Cohort Profile: The Health Outcomes and Measures of the Environment (HOME) Study. Int J Epidemiol 2017;46:24–24. doi:10.1093/ije/dyw006.

[46] Jackson-Browne MS, Papandonatos GD, Chen A, Calafat AM, Yolton K, Lanphear BP, Braun JM. Identifying vulnerable periods of neurotoxicity to triclosan exposure in children. Environ Health Perspect 2018;126:057001. doi:10.1289/EHP2777.

[47] Stacy SL, Eliot M, Etzel T, Papandonatos G, Calafat AM, Chen A, Hauser R, Lanphear BP, Sathyanarayana S, Ye X, et al. Patterns, variability, and predictors of urinary triclosan concentrations during pregnancy and childhood. Environ Sci Technol 2017;51: 6404–13. doi:10.1021/acs.est.7b00325.

[48] Meeker JD, Ferguson KK. Urinary phthalate metabolites are associated with decreased serum testosterone in men, women, and children from NHANES 2011–2012. J Clin Endocrinol Metab 2014;99:4346–52. doi:10.1210/jc.2014-2555.

[49] Hornung RW, Reed LD. Estimation of average concentration in the presence of nondetectable values. Appl Occup Environ Hyg 1990;5:46–51. doi:10.1080/1047322X.1990.10389587.

[50] Larsen K. Creatinine assay by a reaction-kinetic principle. Clin Chim Acta Int J Clin Chem 1972;41:209–17. doi:10.1016/0009-8981(72)90513-x.

[51] Jackson-Browne MS, Papandonatos GD, Chen A, Yolton K, Lanphear BP, Braun JM. Early-life triclosan exposure and parent-reported behavior problems in 8-year-old children. Environ Int 2019;128:446–56. doi:10.1016/j.envint.2019.01.021.

[52] Carroll RJ, Ruppert D, Stefanski LA, Crainiceanu CM. Measurement error in nonlinear models: A modern perspective, Second edition. London: Chapman and Hall/CRC, 2006.

[53] Wechsler D. Manual for the Weschler intelligence scale for children, Third edition (WISC-III). San Antonio, TX: Psychological Corporation, 1991.

[54] Wechsler D. The Wechsler preschool and primary scale of intelligence, Third Edition (WPPSI-III). San Antonio, TX: Psychological Corporation, 2002.

[55] Goldstein S, Naglieri JA, eds. WISC-IV. In: Goldstein S, Naglieri JA, eds. Encyclopedia of child behavior and development. Boston, MA: Springer, 2011.

[56] Werner EF, Braun JM, Yolton K, Khoury JC, Lanphear BP. The association between maternal urinary phthalate concentrations and blood pressure in pregnancy: The HOME Study. Environ Health Glob Access Sci 2015;14:75. doi:10.1186/s12940-015-0062-3.

[57] van der Laan MJ, Polley EC, Hubbard AE. Super learner. Stat Appl Genet Mol Biol 2007;6:25. doi:10.2202/1544-6115.1309.

[58] Benowitz NL, Bernert JT, Caraballo RS, Holiday DB, Wang J. Optimal serum cotinine levels for distinguishing cigarette smokers and nonsmokers within different racial/ethnic groups in the United States between 1999 and 2004. Am J Epidemiol 2009;169:236–48. doi:10.1093/aje/kwn301.

[59] Wechsler D. Wechsler Abbreviated scale of intelligence, Second edition. San Antonio, TX: Psychological Corporation, 1999.

[60] Hintze JL, Nelson RD. Violin plots: A box plot-density trace synergism. Am Stat 1998;52:181. doi:10.2307/2685478.

[61] Tingley D, Yamamoto T, Hirose K, Keele L, Imai K, Trinh M, Woing W. Causal mediation analysis, 2019. URL https://imai.princeton.edu/projects/mechanisms.html.

[62] Baron RM, Kenny DA. The moderator–mediator variable distinction in social psychological research: conceptual, strategic, and statistical considerations. J Pers Soc Psychol 1986;51:1173–82. doi:10.1037/0022-3514.51.6.1173.

[63] Caldwell BM, Bradley RH. The Home Observation for Measurement of the Environment Revisited. Child Adolesc Ment Health 1978;9:25–35. doi:10.1046/j.1475-357X.2003.00073.x.

[64] Braun JM, Hornung R, Chen A, Dietrich KN, Jacobs DE, Jones R, Khoury JC, Liddy-Hicks S, Morgan S, Vanderbeek SB, et al. Effect of residential lead-hazard interventions on childhood blood lead concentrations and neurobehavioral outcomes: A randomized clinical trial. JAMA Pediatr 2018;172:934–42. doi:10.1001/jamapediatrics.2018.2382.

[65] Jones DR, Jarrett JM, Tevis DS, Franklin M, Mullinix NJ, Wallon KL, Derrick Quarles C, Caldwell KL, Jones RL. Analysis of whole human blood for Pb, Cd, Hg, Se, and Mn by ICP-DRC-MS for biomonitoring and acute exposures. Talanta 2017;162:114–22. doi:10.1016/j.talanta.2016.09.060.

[66] Sears CG, Braun JM, Ryan PH, Xu Y, Werner EF, Lanphear BP, Wellenius GA. The association of traffic-related air and noise pollution with maternal blood pressure and hypertensive disorders of pregnancy in the HOME Study Cohort. Environ Int 2018;121: 574–81. doi:10.1016/j.envint.2018.09.049.

[67] Diez Roux AV, Merkin SS, Arnett D, Chambless L, Massing M, Nieto FJ, Sorlie P, Szklo M, Tyroler HA, Watson RL. Neighborhood of residence and incidence of coronary heart disease. N Engl J Med 2001;345:99–106. doi:10.1056/NEJM200107123450205.

[68] R Core Team R: A language and environment for statistical computing. R foundation for statistical computing. Vienna: European Environment Agency, 2020.

[69] Rubin IL, Merrick J. Introduction: Out of Africa. In: Rubin IL, Merrick J, eds. International aspects of environmental health. Public Health: Practices, Methods and Policies. New York: Nova Science, 2016.

[70] Calafat AM, Silva MJ, Reidy JA, Earl Gray L, Samandar E, Preau JL, Herbert AR, Needham LL. Mono-(3-Carboxypropyl) phthalate, a metabolite of Di-n-Octyl phthalate. J Toxicol Environ Health A 2006;69:215–27. doi:10.1080/15287390500227381.

[71] Wallner P, Kundi M, Hohenblum P, Scharf S, Hutter HP. Phthalate metabolites, consumer habits and health effects. Int J Environ Res Public Health 2016;13(7):717. doi:10.3390/ijerph13070717.

[72] Bloom MS, Wenzel AG, Brock JW, Kucklick JR, Wineland RZ, Cruze L, Unal ER, Yucel RM, Jiyessova A, Newman RB. Racial disparity in maternal phthalates exposure; association with racial disparity in fetal growth and birth outcomes. Environ Int 2019;127:473–86. doi:10.1016/j.envint.2019.04.005.

[73] James-Todd TM, Chiu YH, Zota A. Racial/ethnic disparities in environmental endocrine disrupting chemicals and women's reproductive health outcomes: Epidemiological examples across the life course. Curr Epidemiol Rep 2016;3:161–80. doi:10.1007/s40471-016-0073-9.

[74] Varshavsky JR, Zota AR, Woodruff TJ. A novel method for calculating potency-weighted cumulative phthalates exposure with implications for identifying racial/ethnic disparities among U.S. reproductive-aged women in NHANES 2001-2012. Environ Sci Technol 2016;50:10616–24. doi:10.1021/acs.est.6b00522.

[75] Branch F, Woodruff TJ, Mitro SD, Zota AR. Vaginal douching and racial/ethnic disparities in phthalates exposures among reproductive-aged women: National Health and Nutrition Examination Survey 2001-2004. Environ Health Glob Access Sci 2015;14:57. doi:10.1186/s12940-015-0043-6.

[76] Buckley JP, Palmieri RT, Matuszewski JM, Herring AH, Baird DD, Hartmann KE, Hoppin JA. Consumer product exposures associated with urinary phthalate levels in pregnant women. J Expo Sci Environ Epidemiol 2012;22:468–75. doi:10.1038/jes.2012.33.

[77] Zota AR, Shamasunder B. The environmental injustice of beauty: Framing chemical exposures from beauty products as a health disparities concern. Am J Obstet Gynecol 2017;217:418. doi:10.1016/j.ajog.2017.07.020.

[78] Krieger,N. Discrimination and health inequities. Int J Health Serv Plan Adm Eval 2014; 44:643–10. doi:10.2190/HS.44.4.b.

[79] Bailey ZD, Krieger N, Agénor M, Graves J, Linos N, Bassett MT. Structural racism and health inequities in the USA: Evidence and interventions. Lancet Lond Engl 2017;389: 1453–63. doi:10.1016/S0140-6736(17)30569-X.

[80] Parameswaran R, Cardoza K. Melanin on the margins: Advertising and the cultural politics of fair/light/white beauty in India. J Commun Monogr 2009;11:213–74. doi:10.1177/152263790901100302.
[81] Bristor JM, Lee RG, Hunt MR. Race and ideology: African-American images in television advertising. Thousand Oaks, CA: Sage, 1995. URL: https://journals.sagepub.com/doi/abs/10.1177/074391569501400105.
[82] Adibi JJ, Whyatt RM, Williams PL, Caalafat AM, Camann D, Herrick R, et al. Characterization of phthalate exposure among pregnant women assessed by repeat air and urine samples. Environ Health Perspect 2008;116:467.
[83] Braun JM, Smith KW, Williams PL, Calafat AM, Berry K, Ehrlich S, Hauser R. Variability of urinary phthalate metabolite and Bisphenol A concentrations before and during pregnancy. Environ Health Perspect 2012;120:739–45. doi:10.1289/ehp.1104139.
[84] Banks I. Hair matters: Beauty, power, and Black women's consciousness. New York: NYU Press, 2000.
[85] Robinson CL. Hair as Race: Why "good hair" may be bad for Black females. Howard J Commun 2011;22(4):358–76.
[86] Johnson AM, Godsil R, MacFarlane J, Tropp L, Goff PA. The "good hair" study: Explicit and implicit attitudes toward Black women's hair. River Falls, WI: Perception Institute, 2017.
[87] James-Todd T, Fitzgeraald T. Caution: "Acceptable" Black women's hairstyles may harm health. Common Health 2014. URL: https://www.wbur.org/commonhealth/2014/07/14/black-womens-hairstyles-health.
[88] Bristor JM, Gravois Lee R, Hunt MR. Race and ideology: African-American images in television advertising. J Public Policy Marketing 1995;14:48–59. doi:10.1177/074391569501400105.
[89] Harley KG, Kogut K, Madrigal DS, Cardenas M, Vera IA, Meza-Alfaro G, et al. Reducing phthalate, paraben, and phenol exposure from personal care products in adolescent girls: Findings from the HERMOSA intervention study. Environ Health Perspect 2016;124:1600–7. doi:10.1289/ehp.1510514.
[90] Braun JM, Yolton K, Stacy SL, Erar B, Papandonatos GD, Bellinger DC, Lanphear BP, Chen A. Prenatal environmental chemical exposures and longitudinal patterns of child neurobehavior. Neurotoxicology 2017;62:192–9. doi:10.1016/j.neuro.2017.07.027.

Supplemental Material

Characterizing racial disparities in the associations between early life phthalate exposure and child cognition

Table S1. Study sample characteristics of mother-child dyads with follow-up at age 5 and/or 8 years by child race, according to covariates in the full [a] cohort sample compared to the analytic sample, stratified by race: the home study (2003-2006)

	Full Sample [b]		Black		White	
	Analytic Sample	Full Sample	Analytic Sample	Full Sample	Analytic Sample	Full Sample
Variable	N (%)	N (%)	N (%)	N (%)	N (%)	N (%)
Overall	253 (100)	389 (100)	90 (36)	123 (32)	145 (57)	242 (62)
Maternal Age						
<25 years	57 (23)	96 (25)	45 (50)	65 (53)	8 (5)	24 (10)
25 - <35 years	154 (61)	231 (59)	40 (44)	48 (39)	104 (72)	169 (70)
35+ years	42 (17)	62 (16)	5 (6)	10 (8)	33 (23)	49 (20)
Maternal Education						
High School or less	62 (25)	95 (25)	51 (57)	67 (57)	7 (5)	12 (5)
Some College	71 (28)	93 (24)	31 (34)	38 (32)	37 (26)	50 (21)
Completed College	120 (47)	196 (51)	8 (9)	17 (14)	101 (70)	165 (70)
Annual Income						
<$30,000	82 (32)	124 (32)	70 (78)	95 (77)	9 (6)	23 (10)
$30,000 - $75,000	77 (30)	121 (31)	17 (19)	22 (18)	55 (38)	93 (38)
≥$75,000	94 (37)	144 (37)	3 (3)	6 (5)	81 (56)	126 (52)

	Full Sample [b]		Black		White	
	Analytic Sample	Full Sample	Analytic Sample	Full Sample	Analytic Sample	Full Sample
Variable	N (%)	N (%)	N (%)	N (%)	N (%)	N (%)
Maternal Smoking [d]						
Unexposed	78 (31)	89 (31)	5 (6)	5 (5)	66 (56)	76 (45)
Second-Hand Smoking	116 (46)	163 (58)	40 (44)	67 (72)	71 (49)	88 (52)
Active Smoking	29 (11)	31 (11)	45 (50)	21 (23)	8 (6)	5 (3)
Parity						
0	114 (45)	173 (45)	29 (32)	39 (32)	73 (50)	117 (49)
1	79 (31)	126 (33)	29 (32)	43 (36)	46 (32)	79 (33)
2 +	60 (24)	94 (24)	32 (36)	43 (36)	26 (18)	48 (20)
Pre-pregnancy BMI (kg/m2)[e]						
Normal/ Underweight <25	125 (49)	142 (50)	32 (36)	32 (34)	83 (57)	98 (58)
Overweight ≥25 - <30	65 (26)	69 (24)	23 (25)	32 (34)	38 (26)	42 (25)
Obese ≥30	63 (25)	65 (23)	35 (39)	36 (39)	24 (17)	25 (15)
Child Sex						
Male	113 (45)	181 (46)	33 (37)	45 (37)	69 (48)	122 (50)
Female	140 (55)	208 (53)	57 (63)	78 (63)	76 (52)	120 (50)

BMI: Body Mass Index, HOME Study: Health Outcomes and Measures of the Environment Study

[a] Note that values may not sum to the full sample size due to missing information from subsets of the original full sample, percentages reflect columns (e.g., race) within each study sample characteristic

[b] Child race category Other for the analytic sample includes Hispanic (n=6, 33%), Native American (n=5, 28%), Asian and Pacific Islander (n=7, 38%)

[c] Maternal race/ethnicity category Other for the analytic sample includes Hispanic (n=7, 39%), Native American (n=2, 11%), Asian and Pacific Islander (n=3, 17%), Multiple/other race (n=6, 33%)

[a] Maternal smoking during pregnancy estimated based on maternal serum cotinine concentrations during pregnancy. Unexposed smoking exposure defined as having serum cotinine concentrations <0.015ng/mL, second-hand smoking exposure is defined by serum cotinine concentrations between 0.015 and <3.00 ng/mL, and active smoking includes those with serum cotinine concentrations ≥3.00 ng/mL.

[e] Pre-pregnancy BMI (kg/m2) was defined as normal/underweight <25, overweight ≥25-<30, and obese ≥30.

Table S2. Univariate statistics (median, Q1, Q3) of error corrected repeated maternal and childhood urinary concentrations of phthalate metabolites (ng/mL)

Phthalate Metabolite	Non-Hispanic Black (N=90)		Non-Hispanic White (N=145)		Percent Difference Between Non-Hispanic Black and Non-Hispanic White (95% CI)	
	Gestation [a]	Childhood [c]	Gestation	Childhood	Gestation	Childhood
MCPP	1.8 (1.8, 3.5)	11.0 (10.0, 12.4)	2.4 (1.76, 3.5)	12.2 (10.4, 14.2)	7.2 (6.2, 8.3)	9.1 (8.6, 9.6)
MiBP	5.8 (3.7, 7.8)	17.4 (15.7, 19.9)	4.4 (2.51, 7.2)	15.6 (14.8, 19.7)	13 (11, 16)	10 (10, 11)
MBzP	13.0 (7.4, 20.7)	36.7 (28.5, 48.7)	7.8 (4.68, 14.0)	27.3 (21.7, 37.2)	16 (13, 21)	13 (12, 15)
MBP	25.0 (16.4, 43.7)	31.7 (27.5, 37.8)	23.9 (16.63, 35.1)	32.1 (26.8, 37.8)	10 (9.1, 13)	10 (9.3, 11)
MCOP [d]	--	33.9 (30.9, 36.8)	--	35.4 (31.6, 38.3)	--	9.6 (9.2, 10)
MCNP [d]	--	10.8 (9.8, 12.5)	--	11.2 (9.8, 12.3)	--	9.8 (9.3, 10)
ΣDEHP [e]	57.6 (39.3, 113.9)	197.9 (180.5, 223.4)	89.0 (52.8, 214.9)	194.1 (173.1, 213.2)	6.3 (5.0, 8.0)	10 (9.8, 101)
MEP	138.3 (79.8, 397.8)	135.4 (104.3, 204.3)	122.28 (63.4, 242.1)	66.7 (50.9, 96.3)	15 (11, 19)	21 (19, 24)

Q1: 1st quartile, Q3: 3rd quartile

MCPP, mono(3- carboxypropyl) phthalate; MiBP, mono-isobutyl phthalate; MBzP, monobenzyl phthalate; MBP, mono-n-butyl phthalate; MCOP, monocarboxyoctyl phthalate; MCNP, monocarboxynonyl phthalate; ΣDEHP, summary di(2-ethylhexyl) phthalate metabolite measure; MEP, monoethyl phthalate

[a] Repeated maternal urinary phthalate metabolites assessed at 16 and 26 weeks gestation

[c] Repeated child urinary phthalate metabolites assessed at age 1, 2, 3, 4, 5, and 8 years, and average childhood values were based on error corrected average trajectories from ages 1,2,3,4 and 5. Note, phthalate concentrations at age 8 years were not included in average childhood values, and the main outcome of average child FSIQ includes values obtained at age 5 and 8 years.

[d] We did not measure MCNP or MCOP concentrations from maternal urine samples, as the method for these biomarkers had not yet been developed at the time of analysis

[e] Concentrations of ΣDEHP (in ng/mL) were calculated using the following formula: ΣDEHP (ng/mL)=[MECPP (ng/mL) /278 g/mol + MEHHP (ng/mL) /294.3 g/mol + MEOHP (ng/mL) /292.2 g/mol + MEHP (ng/mL) /278.3 g/mol] *278 g/mol.

Table S3. Limits of detection and percent of participants below the value of the limit of detection for repeated maternal and childhood urinary concentrations of phthalate metabolites (ng/mL)

Phthalate		Visit															
		16 Weeks		26 Weeks		1 Year		2 Years		3 Years		4 Years		5 Years		8 Years	
Metabolite	LOD	N	%<LOD	N	%<LOD	N	%<LOD	N	%<LOD	N	%<LOD	N	%<LOD	N	%<LOD	N	%<LOD
MCPP	0.20	252	1.6%	245	3.3%	213	0.0%	188	0.0%	196	1.5%	166	0.6%	202	0.0%	220	0.0%
MiBP [a]	0.30	252	2.8%	245	5.4%	--	--	--	--	--	--	166	0.0%	202	0.5%	220	0.0%
MBzP	0.22	252	1.2%	245	1.6%	213	0.5%	188	0.5%	196	0.5%	166	0.0%	202	0.0%	220	0.5%
MBP [a]	0.60	252	0.0%	245	0.0%	--	--	--	--	--	--	166	0.0%	202	1.5%	220	0.9%
MCOP [b]	0.50	--	--	--	--	213	0.0%	188	0.5%	196	1.5%	166	0.0%	202	1.5%	220	0.0%
MCNP [b]	0.50	--	--	--	--	213	1.4%	188	0.0%	196	4.1%	166	0.0%	202	0.0%	220	0.0%
ΣDEHP [c]	--	--	--	--	--	--	--	--	--	--	--	--	--	--	--	--	--
MEP	0.53	252	0.0%	245	0.0%	213	0.0%	188	0.0%	196	0.0%	166	0.0%	202	0.0%	220	0.0%

LOD: Limit of detection

MCPP, mono(3- carboxypropyl) phthalate; MiBP, mono-isobutyl phthalate; MBzP, monobenzyl phthalate; MBP, mono-n-butyl phthalate; MCOP, monocarboxyoctyl phthalate; MCNP, monocarboxynonyl phthalate; ΣDEHP, summary di(2-ethylhexyl) phthalate metabolite measure; MEP, monoethyl phthalate

[a] We did not measure MiBP or MBP concentrations from childhood urinary samples at ages 1, 2, and 3 years

[b] We did not measure MCNP or MCOP concentrations from maternal urine samples, as the method for these biomarkers had not yet been developed at the time of analysis

[b] Concentrations of ΣDEHP (in ng/mL) were calculated using the following formula: ΣDEHP (ng/mL)=[MECPP (ng/mL) /278 g/mol + MEHHP (ng/mL) /294.3 g/mol + MEOHP (ng/mL) /292.2 g/mol + MEHP (ng/mL) /278.3 g/mol] *278 g/mol.

Table S4. Adjusted [a] direct and indirect effects of the associations between race and child FSIQ at ages 5 or 8 per 10-fold increase in gestational and childhood urinary phthalate metabolite concentrations

	Visit	**N (%) by Race**		**Direct Effect**		**Indirect Effect**	
Metabolite		**Black**	**White**	**β (95% CI)**	**P-value**	**β (95% CI)**	**P-value**
MBzP	1 Year	68 (76)	127 (88)	-8.1 (-13.9, -2.3)	<0.01	0.7 (-0.2, 2.2)	0.15
	2 Years	45 (50)	126 (87)	-7.0 (-12.8, -1.4)	0.01	0.4 (-0.7, 1.8)	0.45
	3 Years	51 (57)	124 (86)	-9.2 (-15.2, -3.4)	<0.01	0.6 (-0.5, 2.1)	0.27
	4 Years	48 (53)	105 (72)	-8.8 (-14.7, -2.9)	<0.01	0.3 (-0.5, 1.4)	0.50
	5 Years	67 (74)	120 (83)	-8.8 (-14.7, -3.0)	<0.01	0.3 (-0.3, 1.3)	0.36
	8 Years	58 (72)	107 (85)	-10.0 (-15.9, -4.4)	<0.01	0.3 (-0.6, 1.5)	0.55
MEP	1 Year	68 (76)	127 (88)	-5.8 (-11.6, 0.3)	0.06	-1.3 (-3.7, 0.8)	0.18
	2 Years	45 (50)	126 (87)	-4.9 (-11.5, 1.6)	0.15	-1.9 (-4.7, 0.7)	0.16
	3 Years	51 (57)	124 (86)	-7.9 (-14.4, -1.3)	0.01	-0.7 (-3.2, 1.9)	0.58
	4 Years	48 (53)	105 (72)	-8.1 (-14.6, -1.3)	0.02	-0.5 (-3.2, 2.2)	0.71
	5 Years	67 (74)	120 (83)	-7.0 (-13.2, -1.0	0.03	-1.1 (-3.6, 1.1)	0.34
	8 Years	58 (72)	107 (85)	-8.2 (-14.9, -1.8)	0.01	-1.5 (-3.5, 0.3)	0.14

MBzP, monobenzyl phthalate; MEP, monoethyl phthalate

[a] Adjusted for maternal age (continuous), pre-pregnancy BMI (continuous), income (continuous), log-10 transformed average gestational cotinine concentration (continuous), and maternal FSIQ scores (continuous)

Table S5. Adjusted [a] associations between average child FSIQ at ages 5 or 8 per 10-fold increase in gestational and childhood MEP urinary phthalate metabolite concentrations

	Time Period	N (%) by Race		Average Adjusted Total Effect (95% CI)	Direct Effect (95% CI)	P-value	Indirect Effect (95% CI)	P-value
		Black	White					
Primary Analysis								
	Gestation	90 (100)	145 (100)	-7.0 (-12.1, -1.8)	-7.0 (-12.1, -2.0)	<0.01	0.1 (-0.4, 0.8)	0.78
	1 Year	68 (76)	127 (88)	-7.0 (-12.1, -1.8)	-5.8 (-11.6, 0.3)	0.06	-1.3 (-3.7, 0.8)	0.18
	2 Years	45 (50)	126 (87)	-7.0 (-12.1, -1.8)	-4.9 (-11.5, 1.6)	0.15	-1.9 (-4.7, 0.7)	0.16
	3 Years	51 (57)	124 (86)	-7.0 (-12.1, -1.8)	-7.9 (-14.4, -1.3)	0.01	-0.7 (-3.2, 1.9)	0.58
	4 Years	48 (53)	105 (72)	-7.0 (-12.1, -1.8)	-8.1 (-14.6, -1.3)	0.02	-0.5 (-3.2, 2.2)	0.71
	5 Years	67 (74)	120 (83)	-7.0 (-12.1, -1.8)	-7.0 (-13.2, -1.0	0.03	-1.1 (-3.6, 1.1)	0.34
	8 Years	58 (72)	107 (85)	-9.6 (-15.5, -3.7)	-8.2 (-14.9, -1.8)	0.01	-1.5 (-3.5, 0.3)	0.14
Adjusted for child sex								
	Gestation	90 (100)	145 (100)	-7.0 (-12.1, -1.9)	-7.0 (-12.2, -1.9)	0.01	0.1 (-0.4, 0.7)	0.79
	1 Year	68 (76)	127 (88)	-7.0 (-12.1, -1.9)	-6.0 (-12.0, 0.4)	0.07	-1.5 (-3.5, 0.4)	0.13
	2 Years	45 (50)	126 (87)	-7.0 (-12.1, -1.9)	-4.0 (-10.4, 2.6)	0.23	-2.2 (-5.1. 0.4)	0.09
	3 Years	51 (57)	124 (86)	-7.0 (-12.1, -1.9)	-6.9 (-13.3, -0.6)	0.03	-1.3 (-3.9, 1.2)	0.33
	4 Years	48 (53)	105 (72)	-7.0 (-12.1, -1.9)	-7.7 (-14.5, -1.0)	0.03	-0.7 (-3.6, 1.8)	0.65
	5 Years	67 (74)	120 (83)	-7.0 (-12.1, -1.9)	-6.8 (-12.7, -0.1)	0.02	-1.5 (-3.9, 0.8)	0.20
	8 Years	58 (72)	107 (85)	-9.6 (-15.5, -3.8)	-9.7 (-15.4, -3.8)	<0.01	0.1 (-0.4, 0.8)	0.75
Adjusted for HOME scores [b]								
	Gestation	90 (100)	145 (100)	-6.7 (-12.1, -1.3)	-6.8 (-12.8, -1.3)	0.02	0.1 (-0.4, 0.8)	0.76
	1 Year	68 (76)	127 (88)	-6.7 (-12.1, -1.3)	-5.6 (-11.7, 0.6)	0.08	-1.5 (-4.0, 0.7)	0.19
	2 Years	45 (50)	126 (87)	-6.7 (-12.1, -1.3)	-4.3 (11.4, 2.1)	0.22	-2.0 (-4.8, 0.6)	0.13
	3 Years	51 (57)	124 (86)	-6.7 (-12.1, -1.3)	-6.8 (-13.4, -0.2)	0.05	-0.9 (-3.7, 1.6)	0.49
	4 Years	48 (53)	105 (72)	-6.7 (-12.1, -1.3)	-4.8 (-12.4, 2.3)	0.19	-0.4 (-3.1, 2.3)	0.76
	5 Years	67 (74)	120 (83)	-6.7 (-12.1, -1.3)	-6.4 (-13.1, -0.2)	0.04	-1.3 (-3.7, 1.1)	0.33
	8 Years	58 (72)	107 (85)	-9.1 (-15.3, -2.9)	-9.2 (-15.5, -2.8)	<0.01	0.1 (-0.4, 0.8)	0.70

Table S5. (Continued)

	Time Period	N (%) by Race		Average Adjusted Total Effect (95% CI)	Direct Effect (95% CI)	P-value	Indirect Effect (95% CI)	P-value
		Black	White					
Adjusted for neighborhood socioeconomic position [c,d]								
	Gestation	88 (100)	142 (100)	-6.1 (-11.7, -0.6)	-6.3 (-11.9, -1.0)	0.03	0.1 (-0.4, 0.7)	0.72
	1 Year	67 (76)	124 (87)	-6.1 (-11.7, -0.6)	-6.1 (-12.3, 0.3)	0.06	-0.9 (-2.9, 1.0)	0.35
	2 Years	45 (51)	123 (87)	-6.1 (-11.7, -0.6)	-4.1 (-10.6, 2.4)	0.21	-1.2 (-3.9,1.3)	0.32
	3 Years	50 (57)	121 (85)	-6.1 (-11.7, -0.6)	-8.6 (-15.7, -1.6)	<0.01	-0.2 (-2.9, 2.7)	0.90
	4 Years	47 (53)	102 (72)	-6.1 (-11.7, -0.6)	-9.0 (-16.4, -1.9)	<0.01	0.2 (-2.5, 2.9)	0.89
	5 Years	66 (75)	117 (82)	-6.1 (-11.7, -0.6)	-7.1 (-13.3, -0.8)	0.02	-0.5 (-2.6, 1.5)	0.63
	8 Years	58 (72)	107 (85)	-10.3 (-16.8, -3.7)	-9.2 (-16.0, -1.9)	0.01	-1.2 (-3.5, 0.5)	0.19
Adjusted for blood lead levels [e]								
	Gestation	90 (100)	145 (100)	-6.9 (-12.1, -1.6)	-7.0 (-12.3, -2.0)	<0.01	0.12 (-0.5, 0.8)	0.68
	1 Year	62 (69)	118 (81)	-6.4 (-12.4, -0.4)	-4.7 (-11.5, 2.4)	0.16	-1.8 (-4.2, 0.2)	0.08
	2 Years	43 (48)	111 (77)	-6.3 (-12.7, 0.0)	-4.6 (-11.7, 2.6)	0.24	-2.2 (-5.4, 0.8)	0.16
	3 Years	47 (52)	105 (72)	-7.0 (-13.3, -0.8)	-7.8 (-14.6, -0.7)	0.03	-0.4 (-3.1, 2.2)	0.77
	4 Years	47 (52)	90 (62)	-7.8 (-14.4, -1.2)	-7.0 (-14.0, 0.6)	0.08	-1.1 (-4.5, 2.2)	0.51
	5 Years	61 (68)	98 (68)	-6.9 (-13.3, -0.4)	-5.7 (-12.4, 1.0)	0.12	-1.2 (-4.2, 1.5)	0.37
	8 Years	54 (67)	83 (66)	-7.7 (-14.0, -1.4)	-6.4 (-12.9, 0.4)	0.07	-1.4 (-3.9, 0.6)	0.19

FSIQ: Full Scale IQ, HOME Scores: Home Observation fort Measurement of the Environment

MEP, monoethyl phthalate

[a] Adjusted for maternal age (continuous), pre-pregnancy BMI (continuous), income (continuous), log-10 transformed average gestational cotinine concentration (continuous), and maternal FSIQ scores (continuous)

[b] Assessment of caregiving environment (Caldwell et al. 1978)

[c] Neighborhood socioeconomic status was assessed using data from the 2000 U.S. Census (Diez Roux et al., 2001). For the census tract of each participant's residence at 20 weeks gestation, a z-score was calculated for the log transformed median household income; percent of households with interest, dividend, or rental income; log transformed median value of housing unit; percent of residents who completed high school; percent of residents who completed college; and percent of residents employed with executive, managerial, or professional occupations. The z-scores for each measure were summed and categorized into terciles, with lower scores representing lower neighborhood socioeconomic status (Diez Roux et al., 2001).

[d] Note that neighborhood SES was only available for a subset of participants (n=230)

[e] Maternal and childhood concentrations of blood lead levels have been log_{10} transformed to satisfy normality assumptions.

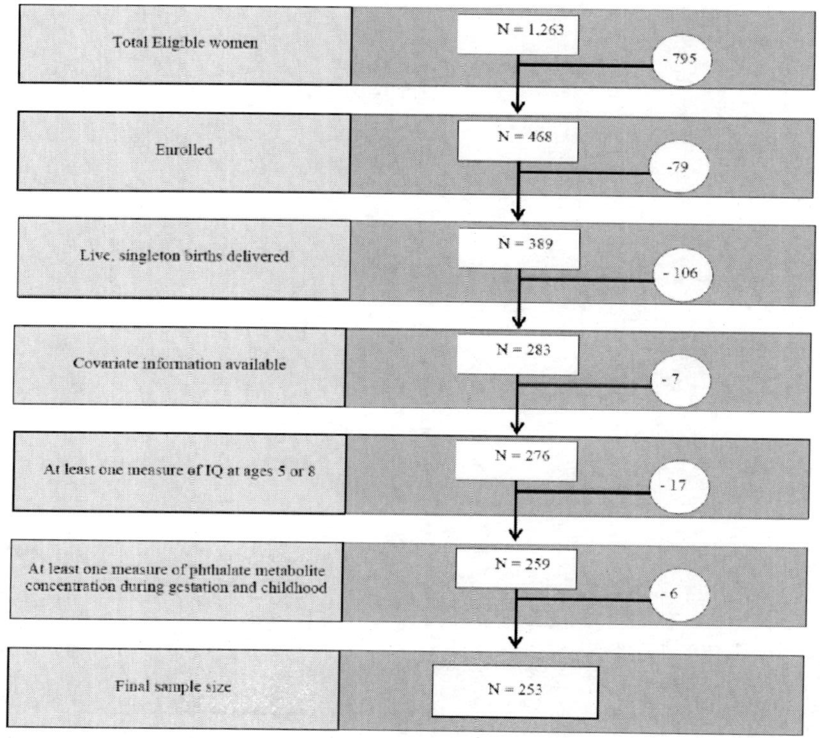

Figure S1. Flow chart of participant selection to final sample size.

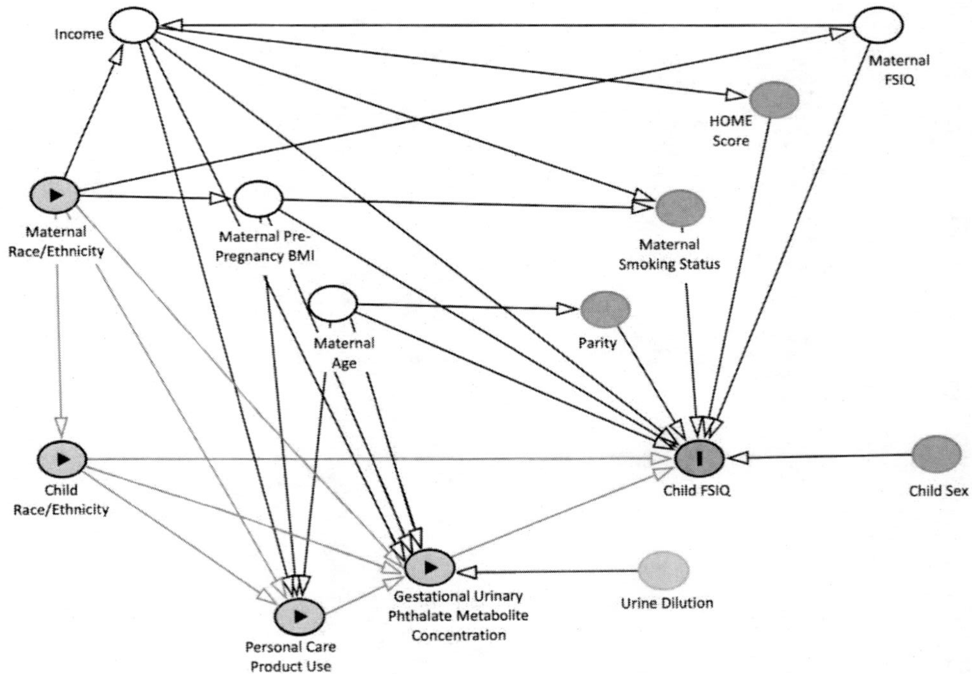

Figure S2. Directed acyclic graph used to select covariates in the association between race and child FSIQ scores through maternal urinary phthalate concentrations.

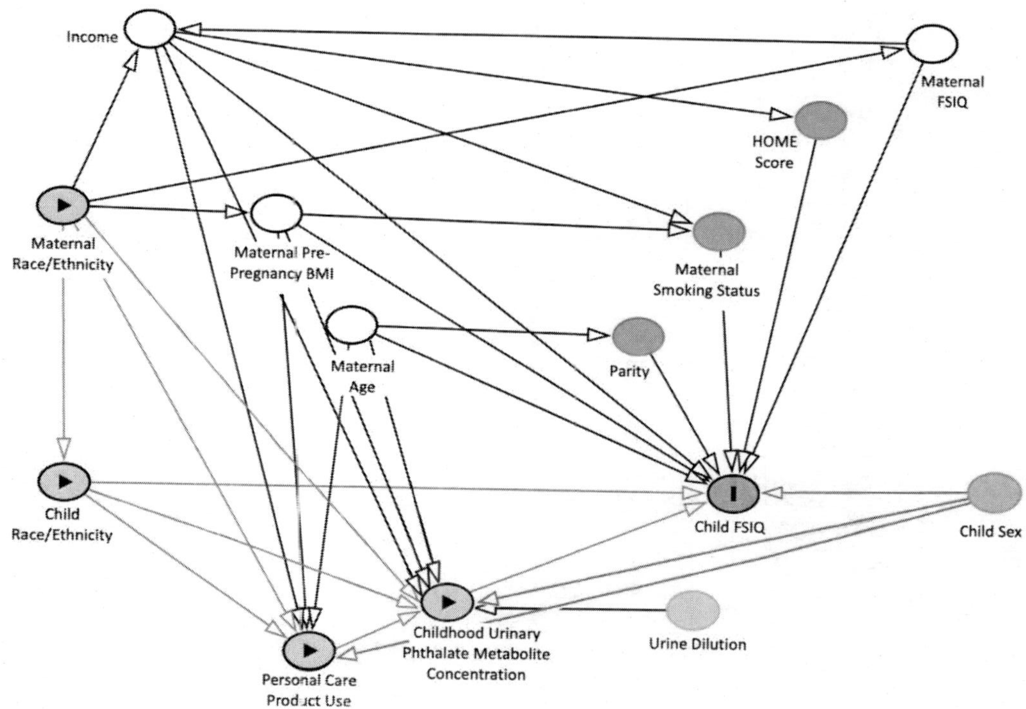

Figure S3. Directed acyclic graph used to select covariates in the association between race and child FSIQ scores through childhood urinary phthalate concentrations.

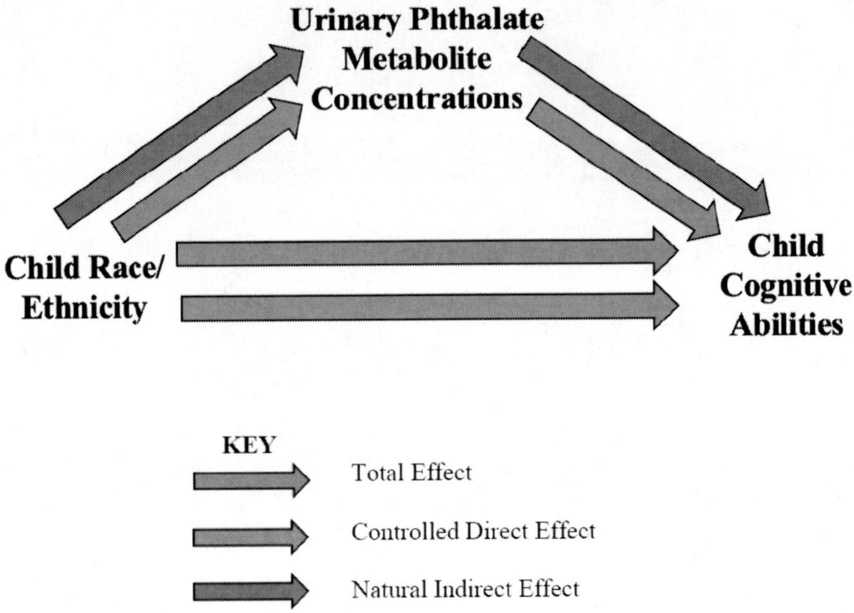

Figure S4. Overview of mediation approach, distinguishing between total, controlled direct, and natural indirect effects.

Chapter 5

Phthalate exposure in children: Assessing knowledge, attitudes and behaviors in families with low socioeconomic status

Rachana Charla*, David Collier, MD, PhD, Melissa Johnson, MPH, Brittany Meier, MA, Andrew Binder, PhD and Katlyn May, MS

Center for Human Health and the Environment, Brody School of Medicine, East Carolina University, Greenville, North Carolina, United States of America

Abstract

Phthalates are a family of synthetic chemicals used in the manufacturing of plastic products, scented products, and personal care products. Exposure to phthalates is a concern as they are considered endocrine disrupting chemicals (EDCs). Here we employed a survey to assess the knowledge, attitudes, and behaviors (KAB) related to phthalates and the use of personal care products that may contain phthalates among 50 parents and caregivers with children no more than five years old at the Brody School of Medicine's Pediatric Outpatient Clinic found at East Carolina University. We found significant relationships between race and product usage with Black respondents more likely to use spray air fresheners, lotions, and candles compared to the non-Black respondents. Additionally, there were significant correlations between income and education level regarding knowledge and recognition of terms like

---

* *Correspondence*: Rachana Charla, BS, Center for Human Health and the Environment, Brody School of Medicine, East Carolina University, Greenville, NC 27834, United States. Email: charlar20@students.ecu.edu, rcharla2468@gmail.com, COLLIERD@ecu.edu.

In: Environmental Health
Editors: I Leslie Rubin and Joav Merrick
ISBN: 979-8-88697-292-4

phthalates. Low socioeconomic status (SES) and lack of knowledge notably affect potential phthalate exposure in children from personal care products as well as cleaning products. Further studies are needed to confirm the significance of these observations.

Introduction

Phthalates are a family of synthetic chemicals that have proven to be harmful endocrine disruptors. An endocrine disrupting chemical (EDC) is a chemical or xenobiotic agent that disrupts some aspect(s) of the endocrine system. Chemicals like phthalates mimic hormones in the body by binding to the same hormone receptors due to the similar shape and structure of the phthalate molecule as the natural hormone. These EDC's act like hormones and can induce potentially harmful effects like interference with reproductive physiology and induction of developmental malformations (1). Phthalates are mainly used as a plasticizer. They are added to plastic products to increase flexibility without compromising the strength or durability of said plastic products, for example plastic containers, water bottles, toys, polyvinyl chloride (PVC) plastics, food packaging, etc. Phthalates are also added to scented products as a solvent used to make fragrances last longer. These scented products include various personal care products like deodorant, shampoo, lotion, perfumes, and air fresheners (2).

Phthalates also act as androgen blocking chemicals. Phthalates prevent androgens like testosterone and dihydrotestosterone (DHT) from mediating their biological effects in the body and have been associated with male reproductive consequences and interference with puberty (3). Animal studies have associated phthalates with numerous reproductive health and developmental problems such as: early onset of puberty, interfering with the natural functioning of the hormone system, interfering with the male reproductive tract development, lower testosterone levels in adolescent males, lower sperm count in adult males, and reproductive and genital defects (4). In humans, phthalates are known to cross the placenta and pose as a health risk for fetuses and infants (5). The most sensitive time period for phthalate exposure and effects is thought to be during weeks 10 to 13 of gestation, a period of extensive reproductive system development (6). One study linked prenatal phthalate exposure to anogenital distance (AGD)—a potential marker of androgenization in male infants (7). This study suggests that phthalates may play a role disrupting endocrine development and the programming of hormonal set points related to metabolism and growth. Finally, a human study with a cohort of over 1,000 mother son pairs found statistically significant correlations between phthalate exposure and delayed language development (8).

Parents who use plastic or personal care products on or around children inadvertently allow phthalates to be absorbed across the skin of infants and young children, circulating their blood stream, and potentially affecting their health. Studies have shown a link between phthalate products and obesity, asthma, and mental and physical development, all in young children with prenatal exposure (9). Columbia University researchers discovered that three-year old children with high prenatal exposure to two types of phthalates, mono-n-butyl phthalate (MnBP) and monoisobutyl phthalate (MiBP), were more likely to have motor delays. Additionally, prenatal exposure to di-n-butyl phthalate (DnBP), diisobutyl phthalate (DiBP), butylbenzyl phthalate (BBzP) may adversely affect child mental, motor, and behavioral development during the preschool (10). However, exposure to phthalates can also impact individuals in the postnatal period and across the lifespan. Personal care products are a source of exposure to potentially endocrine-disrupting chemicals such as phthalates, parabens, triclosan, and benzophenone-3 (BP-3) which are of particular concern for adolescent girls who use such products at a much higher rate compared to adolescent boys (11). While the negative health effects of phthalates are becoming more public, many parents remain unaware of the impacts on children.

Exposures can be oral, e.g., di(2- ethylhexyl) phthalate (DEHP) via phthalate-contaminated food, water and other liquids and in children through mouthing of toys and teethers or dermal, e.g., diethyl phthalate (DEP), via cosmetics and other personal care products. Exposure can also be via inhalation; phthalates volatilize from PVC, nail polish, hair spray, and other phthalate-containing products (12). For children, primary sources of exposure are thought to be PVC-containing plastic products like lunchboxes and backpacks, personal care products, food and food packaging, and background indoor air/dust exposures (13). For infants and children, added skin contact with surfaces and frequent mouthing of fingers and other objects, e.g., plastic utensils and water bottles, may lead to higher phthalate exposures, as might ingestion of phthalates present in breast milk, infant formula, cow's milk or food packaging (14). Phthalates and their potential substitutes, including non-phthalate plasticizers, are ubiquitous in home environments due to their presence in building materials, plastics, and personal care products (15). As a result, exposure to these potentially toxic compounds is nearly universal. The

CDC has measured 13 phthalate metabolites in the urine of participants in the 2003-2004 National Health and Nutrition Examination Survey (NHANES) (16). These findings indicate that phthalate exposure is widespread in the U.S. population. The study also found that non-Hispanic Blacks have higher levels of several phthalate metabolites than non-Hispanic Whites suggesting higher levels of exposure (17). However, understanding which products in the home are associated most strongly with particular exposures and the primary pathways of exposure are unclear. This study aims to assess parental knowledge, attitudes, and behaviors towards phthalates and other EDCS for a more comprehensive look at how exposure occurs in young children.

Our study

A survey comprised of over 80 potential questions spanning knowledge, attitudes, and behaviors (KABs) about phthalates in personal care products were compiled from various studies including the Toddler's Exposure to SVOCs in the Indoor Environment (TESIE) study and North Carolina Survey on Human Health and the Environment. The TESIE study questionnaire provided a baseline understanding for asking comprehensive environmental exposure questions (18). The North Carolina Survey on Human Health & the Environment provided data and questions about statewide environmental health literacy and baseline data for respondents to be compared to (19). Select findings from the current study were compared to those present in the larger North Carolina Survey on Human Health and the Environment, to highlight the potential differences between local participants and those throughout the state. Although the survey used in this study contained questions from established and developed surveys, the survey was created exclusively for this study and was peer reviewed by the survey developers of and North Carolina Survey on Human Health and the Environment. Questions were chosen from these surveys based on ability to assess KABs and applicability to the survey population.

Participants were recruited from the East Carolina University Brody School of Medicine's Pediatric Outpatient Clinic. Approximately 80% of the patients in this clinic receive Medicaid, about 60% were Black, 25% White, and 15% Latino. Inclusion criteria included a child less than or equal to five years old, presenting with a parent or guardian that they live with and English speaking. Candidates meeting inclusion criteria were identified by the attending physicians and then approached by the research team for obtaining informed written consent and survey administration.

The final survey included 80 items, spanning product usage, KABs, and demographics. After providing informed consent, respondents were asked three demographic questions related to inclusion criteria (e.g., "What is your relationship to the child?"). These were followed by a series of yes/no (e.g., "Does your child use cups, sippy cups, or cups with straws?"), multiple response (e.g., "If yes, do/did you use glass, metal, silicone, or plastic sippy and straw cups?"), Likert-type (e.g., "In the past month, how often do you light candles in your home?"), and open-ended questions (e.g., "If so, what brand/type of candle do you use most often?"). Respondents also received 10 questions regarding chemicals in products (e.g., Are you concerned about the chemicals in your home affecting your health?"). The survey concluded with nine demographic questions regarding oneself, one's child, and one's partner, if applicable. These related to gender, race, ethnicity, household composition, education, and income (e.g., "What is your current yearly income?")

The majority of surveys were administered using Qualtrics, an online survey software, with an investigator reading the questions aloud to participants. Due to technical difficulties, some surveys were administered on paper with an investigator in the room reading questions aloud with participants and responses being input into Qualtrics at a later date. Participants received a $20 monetary compensation for their time. This study was approved by the University Medical Center Institutional Revies Board (UMCIRB #21-000265).

Data analysis

SPSS v27 was used to conduct statistical analyses. While cleaning data, variables were recoded as needed to ensure consistency. Text responses were manually cleaned and assessed to determine response. Descriptive statistics were obtained for demographic and other categorical responses, i.e., nominal measurements, as well as relative use variables, e.g., how often do you…?; i.e., ordinal scales. To compare categorical variables, contingency tables were developed. Due to the sample size and distribution of data, cell counts did not always reach expected values. To account for this, two-sided Fisher's exact tests were employed.

Our findings

A total of 50 subjects completed surveys (see Table 1). Most respondents identified as Black (62.0%), a majority (56.0%) reported their income was $29,000 or less.

Table 1. Respondents' demographics

	Number of Respondents (%) (n = 50)
Relationship to Child*	
Biological Mother	39 (78.0)
Biological Father	8 (16.0)
Other	3 (6.0)
Ethnicity	
Hispanic/Latino/Spanish	9 (18.0)
Not Hispanic/Latino/Spanish	41 (82.0)
Race**	
American Indian/Alaskan Indian	0 (0.0)
Asian	1 (2.0)
Black/African American	31 (62.0)
Hawaiian Native/Pacific Islander	1 (2.0)
White	14 (28.0)
Other	4 (8.0)
Highest Level of Education Completed	
Less than High School	1 (2.0)
High School/GED/Equivalent	15 (30.0)
Some College (No Degree)	18 (36.0)
Associates Degree	8 (16.0)
Bachelor's Degree	5 (10.0)
Graduate School	3 (6.0)
Resides with a Partner***	
Yes	29 (59.2)
No	20 (40.8)
Partner's Relationship to Child***	
Biological Parent	28 (96.6)
Other	1 (3.4)
Partner's Highest Level of Education Completed***	
Less than High School	1 (3.6)
High School/GED/Equivalent	13 (46.4)
Some College (No Degree)	4 (14.3)
Associates Degree	4 (14.3)
Bachelor's Degree	2 (7.1)
Graduate School	4 (14.3)

	Number of Respondents (%) (n = 50)
Income	
Less than $10,000	11 (22.0)
$10,000-19,000	7 (14.0)
$20,000-29,000	10 (20.0)
$30,000-39,000	8 (16.0)
$40,000-49,000	3 (6.0)
$50,000-59,000	3 (6.0)
$60,000-69,000	3 (6.0)
$70,000-79,000	1 (2.0)
$80,000-89,000	0 (0.0)
$90,000-99,000	0 (0.0)
$100,000 or more	4 (8.0)
Socioeconomic Status***	
Lower SES	28 (56.0)
Middle SES	18 (36.0)
Upper SES	4 (8.0)

* Other responses include aunt, grandmother, and great grandmother. ** Respondents were instructed to select "all that apply," potentially resulting in total response rates over 100%. *** SES is based upon data from the Pew Research Center (20). Lower SES = < $29,000, Middle SES = $30,000-99,000, and Upper SES = > $100,000.

Note. Missing responses are not included in overall calculations.

Based on information from Pew Research Center, the following socioeconomic statuses (SES) were defined by annual income: Lower SES: < $29,000, Middle SES: $30,000-99,000, and Upper SES: > $100,000 (20). The majority of children were younger than 13 months old (52.0%) and identified as Black (64.0%) (Table 2). Black respondents (64.5%) were significantly more likely than non-Black respondents (42.1%) to be in the low income bracket; $p = .023$ and non-Black (78.9%) respondents are significantly more likely to have a spouse/partner in their home than Black respondents (46.7%); $p = .037$.

Recognition of the terms "endocrine disruptors," $p = .016$, or "phthalates," $p = .033$, increase with SES. Respondents with lower levels of education were significantly more likely to not recognize the terms "endocrine disruptors," $p < .001$, "phthalates," $p = .019$, or "parabens," $p = 0.41$ than those who received higher levels of education. Consistent with these findings, respondents with lower education levels were more likely to have no chemical concerns, though this relationship fell short of statistical significance, $p = .395$. Similarly, there

Table 2. Children's demographics

	Number of Respondents (%) (n = 50)
Gender*	
Female	28 (56.0)
Male	22 (44.0)
Age (in months)**	
< 13 months	26 (52.0)
13 or more months	24 (48.0)
Ethnicity	
Hispanic/Latino/Spanish	8 (16.0)
Not Hispanic/Latino/Spanish	42 (84.0)
Race***	
American Indian/Alaskan Indian	0 (0.0)
Asian	0 (0.0)
Black/African American	32 (64.0)
Hawaiian Native/Pacific Islander	0 (0.0)
White	15 (30.0)
Other	7 (14.0)
Feeding Type (n = 26)	
Breast Milk – Breast Fed	4 (15.4)
Breast Milk – Bottle Fed	3 (11.5)
Formula – Bottle Fed	19 (73.1)

* Respondents were provided an "other" gender response. In the current sample, no respondents selected this. ** For the current sample, children ranged in age from 0- to 108-months-old (M = 19.16, SD = 19.72). *** Respondents were instructed to select "all that apply," potentially resulting in total response rates over 100%.
Note. Missing responses are not included in the overall response rates.

were no significant relationships between race of SES and perceived avoidance of chemicals or concerns about harm to oneself or one's child (see Table 3). Non-Black respondents' recognition of the terms "endocrine disruptors," "phthalates," "parabens" did not significantly differ from those of Black respondents. Overall, respondents were more familiar with the term "parabens" (40.0%) than with "endocrine disruptors" (14.0%) or "phthalates" (20.0%) (see Table 4).

Thirty-six percent of respondents reported using spray air fresheners daily, while 26.0% respondents reported usage as never. While 36.0% of respondents reported using plug in air fresheners daily similar to spray air fresheners, 38.0% of respondents reported never using plug in air fresheners (see Table 4). There were no significant relationships between familial SES and usage of spray air fresheners, p = .212, or plug in air fresheners,

$p = .362$. However, when comparing families who identified as Black versus families who identified as non-Black, families identifying as Black used significantly more personal care products focusing on improving household smell. Black respondents were shown to use more spray air fresheners, $p = .047$. Black respondents' use of scented candles was also significant as Black respondents used candles for longer periods of time than non-Black respondents; non-Black respondents were significantly more likely to never use candles than Black respondents, $p = .018$ (see Table 5). There were also significant differences in the usage of select personal care products, such as lotion (see Table 6).

Table 3. Opinions about chemicals

Respondents find chemicals in their homes to be _____:	Number of Respondents (%) (n = 50)				
	Not at all	**A little**	**Somewhat**	**Very**	**Extremely**
Concerning for their child's health	23 (46.0)	8 (16.0)	12 (24.0)	3 (6.0)	4 (8.0)
Concerning for their own health	29 (58.0)	4 (8.0)	9 (18.0)	6 (12.0)	2 (4.0)
Avoidable	5 (10.0)	3 (6.0)	12 (24.0)	22 (44.0)	8 (16.0)

Table 4. Chemical name recognition

	Number of Respondents (%) (n = 50)	
	Yes	**No**
Endocrine Disruptors	7 (14.0)	43 (86.0)
Phthalates	10 (20.0)	40 (80.0)
Parabens	20 (40.0)	30 (60.0)

Table 5. Frequency of product use

	Number of Respondents (%)				
	Never	**Once a month**	**Once a week**	**More than twice a week**	**Daily**
Nail Polish (n = 44)	38 (86.4)	6 (13.6)	0 (0.0)	0 (0.0)	0 (0.0)
Body Wash (n = 44)	5 (11.4)	0 (0.0)	2 (4.5)	11 (25.0)	26 (59.1)
Lotion (n = 44)	5 (11.4)	0 (0.0)	1 (2.2)	10 (22.7)	28 (63.6)
Hand Sanitizer (n = 45)	28 (62.2)	0 (0.0)	1 (2.2)	4 (8.9)	12 (26.7)

Table 5. (Continued)

	Number of Respondents (%)				
	Never	**Once a month**	**Once a week**	**More than twice a week**	**Daily**
2-in-1 Shampoo and Conditioner (n = 46)	26 (56.5)	7 (15.2)	6 (13.0)	4 (8.7)	3 (6.5)
Shampoo (n = 45)	15 (33.3)	9 (20.0)	7 (15.6)	8 (17.8)	6 (13.3)
Conditioner (n = 45)	23 (51.1)	8 (17.8)	6 (13.3)	3 (6.7)	5 (11.1)
Plastic food containers (for storing food; n = 49)	28 (57.1)	2 (4.1)	3 (6.1)	9 (18.4)	7 (14.3)
Plastic food containers (for heating food; n = 49)	31 (63.3)	2 (4.1)	4 (8.2)	5 (10.2)	7 (14.3)
Spray Air Fresheners (n = 50)	13 (26.0)	2 (4.0)	12 (24.0)	5 (10.0)	18 (36.0)
Plug-in Air Fresheners (n = 50)	19 (38.0)	7 (14.0)	4 (8.0)	2 (4.0)	18 (36.0)
Car Air Fresheners (n = 49)	26 (53.1)	9 (18.4)	2 (4.1)	1 (2.0)	11 (22.4)

Note. Missing and "other" responses are not included in the overall response rates.

Table 6. Race and product usage

		Number of Respondents (%)**				
		Never	**Once a month**	**Once a week**	**More than twice a week**	**Daily**
Lotion*	Black or African American	3 (10.7)	0 (0.0)	1 (3.6)	2 (7.1)	22 (78.6)
	Not Black or African American	2 (12.5)	0 (0.0)	0 (0.0)	8 (50.0)	6 (37.5)
Shampoo**	Black or African American	11 (37.9)	7 (24.1)	7 (24.1)	3 (10.3)	1 (3.4)
	Not Black or African American	4 (25.0)	2 (12.5)	0 (0.0)	5 (31.3)	5 (31.3)
Conditioner***	Black or African American	13 (44.8)	7 (24.1)	6 (20.7)	2 (6.9)	1 (3.4)
	Not Black or African American	10 (62.5)	1 (6.3)	0 (0.0)	1 (6.3)	4 (25.0)

* p = .005.
** p = .007.
*** p = .029.
Note. Two-sided Fisher's exact tests were used to obtain reported p-values. Missing responses are not included in the overall response rates.

Washing children's hands is an important behavior to minimize exposures to some EDCs. We found that neither race, $p = .109$, nor SES was predictive of handwashing, $p = .423$. Additionally, relationship to the child did not predict handwashing frequency in this sample. Biological mothers report washing children's hands with soap and water more frequently than biological fathers, although this relationship fell short of statistical significance; $p = .462$.

Table 7. North Carolina questions

In the past 12 months, have you _____?	Number of Respondents in ECU Sample (%) (n = 50)	Number of Respondents in NC Sample (%) (n = 1505)
Used a water filter	25 (50.0)	940 (62.9)
Read food labels	35 (70.0)	1185 (79.3)
Avoided insecticides	31 (62.0)	861 (57.6)

Finally, select items were compared to those included in a North Carolina Survey on Human Health & the Environment that surveyed a representative sample of the North Carolina general population. There were no significant differences in reported water filter use (50.0% vs 62.9%), reading food labels (70.0% vs 79.3%) or avoiding insecticide use (62.0% vs 57.6%) between this study cohort and the larger cohort described (18), respectively (see Table 7).

Discussion

Recruiting caregivers at ECU's Pediatric Clinic resulted in a demographically diverse study cohort allowing us to examine the relationships between race, education, and income on knowledge, attitudes, and behaviors specifically related to phthalates and EDCs in general. We hypothesized that families with low education levels were less likely to recognize terms like "phthalates" and "parabens." The linkage between education and health literacy has been established and based on findings published by the National Institute of Environmental Health Science, environmental health literacy is critical to understanding the publics knowledge of environmental and how that contributes to health disparities (19). Indeed, both lower educational attainment and lower income were associated with a lack of recognition of the terms "endocrine disruptors" and "phthalates." Additionally, education attainment was associated with recognition of "parabens" with higher recognition among respondents who obtained higher levels of education.

We also hypothesized that families with low SES backgrounds were more likely to use highly scented personal care and cleaning products such as spray air fresheners, plug in air fresheners, and candles. The likelihood that respondents have children in the home or may live in low-income housing that emits strong odors increases the likelihood of using scented personal care products to make the home feel clean and get rid of any persisting odors. While we did not find a significant relationship between SES and use of spray air fresheners, plug-ins and candles, Black respondents were significantly more likely to use all these products. Similarly, The Taking Stock Study surveyed 357 women reporting and average usage of eight products a day among respondents, with some using up to 30 products daily. Researchers compared product use among Black, Hispanic/Latinx, Asian, and White women, noting for 28 of the products, use varied significantly by race/ethnicity, with the largest differences seen between Black and White women. More specifically, Black women reported using a higher number of hair products with 70 percent of women preferring scented over unscented options (20). Hence race may represent a risk factor for exposure to phthalates from these classes of products. Race, SES, and parental gender were not predictive of frequency of washing children's hands. Perhaps further exploration with a larger sample would yield different results.

Many questionnaires, survey-based studies and predictive models of phthalate exposure show poor correlation with more direct measures of exposure such as measuring urinary concentrations of phthalate metabolites. Phthalates have a relatively short half-life which creates inaccuracy when calculating exposures and from where (21). Many research projects focus on phthalates health impacts by collecting urine samples and employing surveys to collect data on 24-hour potential exposures. Many of these surveys are not conclusive enough to understand where exposures are coming from. These surveys ask few questions about overall behaviors and focus on behaviors on the day of urine testing to find potential phthalate exposures that may show up in the urine. The survey used in this study aims to better understand overall behavior and knowledge of parents and how this relates to potential exposures for the children. Other studies that involve surveys such as the TESIE study have asked relatively similar questions surrounding knowledge attitudes. Compared to those surveys, the results from our questionnaire were similar. Several questions from the North Carolina Survey on Human Health and the Environment, distributed around North Carolina were used to provide a baseline understanding of exposure and behaviors. The behaviors aligned as respondents followed similar trends.

The most significant finding from the survey was the relationship between race and product usage. Black respondents were more likely to use lotion daily compared to their non-Black counterparts, but less likely to use shampoo and conditioner daily compared to their non-Black counterparts. Hair and skin care products are often used on a preferential basis that varies from respondent to respondent and as a result gauging potential phthalate exposure based on brand usage is not possible. Understanding that product usage varies significantly by race due to unique hair and skin needs calls for further research into those potential phthalate exposures even more so among children of different races. Lotion proves especially notable as daily use of a dermal product increases child exposure significantly. The little use of shampoo and conditioner may be safer as the scalp tends to absorb products much faster than other parts of the body.

Another significant relationship was identified between education, SES, and recognition of terms. The recognition of terms including "endocrine disruptors," "parabens," and "phthalates," were asked among participants. The term "parabens" had the highest overall recognition among participants. The specificity of "endocrine disruptors" and "phthalates" was lost among respondents. The education and SES background supported an original claim that respondents with higher education and higher SES were more likely to recognize these terms than respondents with lower education and lower SES. This signals a need for more comprehensive ways to teach environmental health literacy for parents with lower education levels and lower SES backgrounds. A better understanding around potential environmental harms for their children can help parents identify what products including toys, cleaning care, and personal care products have low potential exposures as well as a lower cost. Keeping this in consideration increases accessibility as well as inclusion when reporting such statistics and behaviors.

For future studies, a revision of the survey and collection of more data by giving the revised survey to families with higher SES background will contribute to a better understanding of the scope of SES on knowledge, attitudes and behaviors surrounding phthalates in personal care products. Additionally, focusing on access to phthalate free products and SES must be analyzed as cost is a major factor impacting accessibility. Moving forward, an interventional study that involves collecting urine samples can allow for stronger evidence to support or oppose hypothesis and correlations between behavior and tangible phthalate exposures in children as well as providing respondents with greater educational intervention to increase health literacy might be a more effective study.

Strengths and weaknesses

Our survey was IRB approved and surveyed a clinical population allowing us to better understand how parents view environmental toxins in general as well as what behaviors might contribute to increased phthalate exposure. Although our survey was not validated, it was able to capture frequency and EDC exposure as well as assessing KAB for our respective population with parental interest. All 50 respondents surveyed fully completed the survey which led to a high participation rate. There was no selection bias in who was able to participate provided they met the base requirement. Despite a lack of funding and short timeline, 50 participants were surveyed and compensated through a $1,000 grant from ECU's Undergraduate Research Creative Awards. The small sample size with only 50 participants greatly affected the ability to make generalizable claims that apply to phthalate exposure in the home.

In future studies, the specificity of questions regarding frequency of usage of plug in, car and spray air fresheners need to be made clearer to get a more accurate understanding of behaviors that increase exposures. More specifically, questions need to be geared towards the product focusing on frequency of changing out plug in air fresheners and how many plug-in air fresheners are found around the home. The lack of specificity around different products like plug in air fresheners and candles may have contributed to inexact data surrounding potential phthalate exposures. Further questions need to be made to gauge exact usage of dermal personal care products like lotions and shampoos in order to better understand how race affects exposures in children. Many children who identified as Black had more specific skin and hair care routines leading to more potential exposure with more chemically based products. This phenomenon needs to be better explored asking questions about what types of lotions and hair care products are used and the knowledge surrounding those products and their behaviors. Additionally, some of the knowledge-based questionnaires led to mixed understandings of chemical concerns as some question's presets trivialized yes or no answers over multiple answers. More specifically, the question asking about concerns, e.g., Are you concerned that chemicals used in the products you buy might affect your child's health?, conflicted with the multiple answer question asking what specific chemicals parents were concerned about.

In the future, letting the respondent have more control on how they answer questions without giving away the goal of the survey is necessary as response bias caused answers to change.

Breaking the Cycle

The excess usage of phthalates and lack of knowledge surrounding its effects has contributed to a cycle of exposure that disproportionately affects people of color and those with lower economic mobility. The solution is simple, purchase and use phthalate free products. However, these phthalate free products are more expensive and are harder to access, especially for people in lower income communities. When breaking down the impacts of phthalates on infants and young children among different ethnicities and socio-economic status, we gain a greater understanding of how the role of race, socioeconomic status, education etc. influences exposure to phthalate.

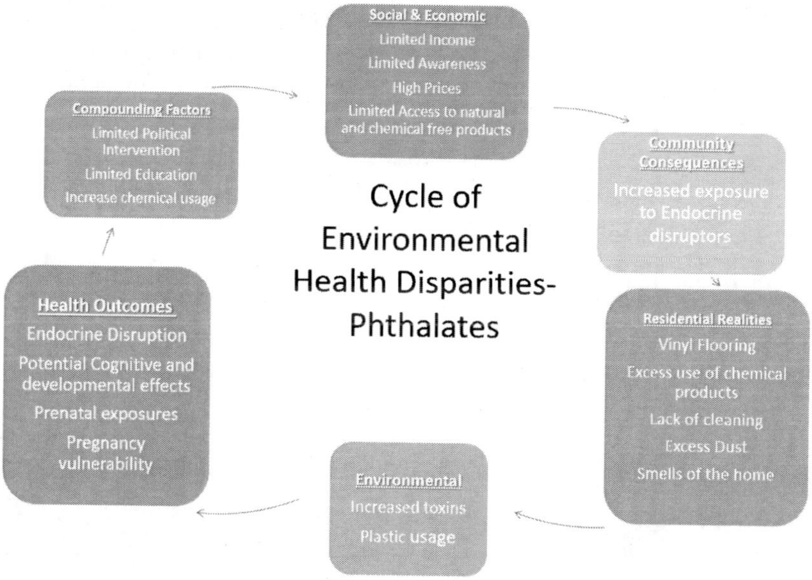

Figure 1. Cycle of environmental health disparities and phthalates.

Understanding what perpetuates the cycle is the key to breaking the cycle. For phthalate exposure in young children, at home behaviors may contribute the most to direct exposure. The use of plastic plates, utensils, water bottles, and other single use plastics around the home contribute greatly to potential exposures, as well as personal care products like lotions, shampoos, and air fresheners. Additionally, scented products used around the home to alleviate undesirable odors can greatly contribute to phthalate exposure in children. These products are frequently used due to convenience and cost, which drives consumer habits and in turn affect exposure. The intersection of race and product use greatly influences potential phthalate exposure in children, as Black children have an increased use of dermal products on the skin.

In order to break this cycle, increasing education and awareness about chemical pollutants found in every day products ensures consumer literacy. This knowledge can affect consumer habits and hopefully create direct change. Realistically, the discrepancies between cost make it hard for parents to responsibly save money while being conscious about chemical exposures.

Breaking the cycle of phthalate exposure requires changes from the government, large corporations, and individual consumers to create lasting impacts. The simplest changes individuals can make include limiting plastic consumption as well as buying products that exclusively state phthalate free with the understanding that this is a worthwhile investment as the higher cost may result in higher quality products with less harmful chemicals. Systematic changes instituted by both the government and large corporations must be made to increase transparency surrounding indoor chemical exposure. More specifically relating to phthalate exposure, changes must be made around phthalate usage and policy in plastic, scented, and personal care products as well as product labeling.

Acknowledgments

Research reported in this publication was supported by the National Institute of Environmental Health Sciences of the National Institutes of Health under Award Number P30ES025128. The content is solely the responsibility of the authors and does not necessarily represent the official views of the National Institutes of Health.

References

[1] Pell T, Eliot M, Chen A, Lanphearc BP, Yolton K, Sathyanarayana S, Braun JM. Parental concern about environmental chemical exposures and children's urinary concentrations of phthalates and phenols. J Pediatrics 2017;186:138–44.

[2] Dutta S, Haggerty DK, Rappolee DA, Ruden DM. Phthalate exposure and long-term epigenomic consequences: A review. Front Genetics 2020;11:405.
[3] Hlisníková H, Petrovičová I, Kolena B, Šidlovská M, Sirotkin A. Effects and mechanisms of phthalates' action on reproductive processes and reproductive health: A literature review. Int J Environ Res Public Health 2020;17(18):6811.
[4] Diamanti-Kandarakis E, Bourguignon JP, Giudice LC, Hauser R, Prins GS, Soto AM, Zoeller RT, Andrea C Gore AC. Endocrine-disrupting chemicals: an endocrine society scientific statement. Endocr Rev 2009;30:293–342.
[5] Kamai EM, McElrath TF, Ferguson KK. Fetal growth in environmental epidemiology: mechanisms, limitations, and a review of associations with biomarkers of non-persistent chemical exposures during pregnancy. Environ Health 2019;18:43.
[6] Qian Y, Shao H, Ying X, Huang W, Hua Y. The endocrine disruption of prenatal phthalate exposure in mother and offspring. Front Public Health 2020;83:66.
[7] Swan SH, Main KM, Liu F, Stewart SL, Kruse RL, Calafat AM, Mao CS, Redmon JB, Ternand CL, Sullivan S, Teague JL, Study for Future Families Research Team. Decrease in anogenital distance among male infants with prenatal phthalate exposure. Environ Health Perspect 2009;113:1056–61.
[8] Bornehag, CG, Lindh, C, Reichenberg, A, Wikström, S, Unenge Hallerback, M, Evans, SF, Sathyanarayana, S, Barrett, ES, Nguyen, RHN., Bush, NR, & Swan, SH. Association of prenatal phthalate exposure with language development in early childhood. JAMA Pediatr 2018;172:1169–76.
[9] Swan SH. Environmental phthalate exposure in relation to reproductive outcomes and other health endpoints in humans. Environ Res 2008;108:177–84.
[10] Meeker JD, Sathyanarayana S, Swan SH. Phthalates and other additives in plastics: human exposure and associated health outcomes. Philos Trans R Soc Lond B Biol Sci 2009;364(1526):2097-113.
[11] Ginsberg G, Ginsberg J, Foos B. Approaches to children's exposure assessment: case study with diethylhexylphthalate (DEHP). Int J Environ Res Public Health 2016;13:670.
[12] National Center for Health Statistics (NCHS). National health and nutrition examination survey data. Hyattsville, MD: US Department of Health and Human Services, Centers for Disease Control and Prevention, 2003-2004.
[13] Zota AR, Calafat AM, Woodruff TJ. Temporal trends in phthalate exposures: Findings from the National Health and Nutrition Examination Survey, 2001-2010. Environ Health Perspect 2014;122(3):235-41.
[14] Braun JM, Sathyanarayana S, Hauser R. Phthalate exposure and children's health. Curr Opin Pediatr 2013;25(2):247–54.
[15] Harley KG, Kogut K, Madrigal DS, Cardenas M, Vera IA, Meza-Alfaro G, She J, Gavin Q, Zahedi R, Bradman, A, Eskenazi B, Kimberly LP. Reducing phthalate, paraben, and phenol exposure from personal care products in adolescent girls: findings from the HERMOSA intervention study. Environ Health Perspect 2013;124(10):1600–7.
[16] Whyatt RM, Liu X, Rauh, VA, Calafat AM, Just AC, Hoepner L, Diaz D, Quinn J, Adibi J, Perera FP, Factor-Litvak P. Maternal prenatal urinary phthalate metabolite

concentrations and child mental, psychomotor and behavioral development at age three years. Environ Health Perspect 2012;120(2):290-5.
[17] Hammel SC, Levasseur JL, Hoffman K, Phillips AL, Lorenzo AM, Calafat AM, Webster TF, and Heather M. Stapleton HM. Children's exposure to phthalates and non-phthalate plasticizers in the home: The TESIE study. Environ Int 2019;132:105061.
[18] Finn S, O'Fallon L. The emergence of environmental health literacy-from its roots to its future potential. Environ Health Perspect 2019;125(4):495–501.
[19] Dodson RE, Cardona B, Zota AR, Robinson Flint J, Navarro S, Shamasunder B. Personal care product use among diverse women in California: Taking Stock Study. J Expo Sci Environ Epidemiol. 2021;31(3):487-502.
[20] Binder AR, May K. Public views on environmental health topics in NC. Raleigh, NC: Center Human Health and Environment, 2021.
[21] Kochhar R. Are you in the American middle class? find out with our income calculator. Washington, DC: Pew Research Center, 2021.
[22] Genuis SJ, Beesoon S, Lobo RA, Birkholz D. Human elimination of phthalate compounds: blood, urine, and sweat (BUS) study. Scientific World Journal 2012;2012:615068.
[23] Daniel L, Michot M, Esvan M, Guérin P, Chauvet G, Pelé F. Perceptions, knowledge, and practices concerning indoor environmental pollution of parents or future parents. Int J Environ Res Public Health 2020;17(20):7669.
[24] Watkins DJ, Eliot M, Sathyanarayana S, Calafat AM, Yolton K, Lanphear BP, Braun J M. Variability and predictors of urinary concentrations of phthalate metabolites during early childhood. Environ Sci Technol 2014;48(15):8881–90.
[25] Koniecki D, Wang R, Moody RP, Zhu J. Phthalates in cosmetic and personal care products: Concentrations and possible dermal exposure. Environ Res 2011;111(3):329–36.
[26] Pacyga DC, Sathyanarayana S, Strakovsky RS. Dietary predictors of phthalate and bisphenol exposures in pregnant women. Adv Nutr 2014;10(5):803–15.
[27] Parlett LE, Calafat AM, Swan SH. Women's exposure to phthalates in relation to use of personal care products. J Expo Sci Environ Epidemiol 2013;23(2):97–206.
[28] Whyatt RM, Liu X, Rauh, VA, Calafat AM, Just AC, Hoepner L, Diaz D, Quinn, J, Adibi, J, Perera, FP, & Factor-Litvak, P. Maternal prenatal urinary phthalate metabolite concentrations and child mental, psychomotor and behavioral development at age three years. Environ Health Perspect 2012;120(2):290-5.
[29] Fisher JS. Environmental anti-androgens and male reproductive health: Focus on phthalates and testicular dysgenesis syndrome. Reprod 2004;127(3):305-15.
[30] Sathyanarayana S, Karr CJ, Lozano P, Brown E, Calafat AM, Liu F, Swan SH. Baby care products: possible sources of infant phthalate exposure. Pediatrics 2008;121(2):e260-8.

Chapter 6

Comparison of neighborhood deprivation index and food desert status as environmental predictors of early childhood obesity

Shannon C Conrey[1,2], PhD, Allison R Burrell[1,2], BSN, Cole Brokamp[1,3], PhD, Rachel M Burke[4], PhD, Sarah C Couch[5], PhD, RD, Liang Niu[1], PhD, Claire P Mattison[4,6], MPH, Daniel C Payne[7], PhD, Mary A Staat[1,2], MD, MPH and Ardythe L Morrow[1,2,*], PhD

[1]University of Cincinnati College of Medicine, Department of Environmental and Public Health Sciences, Cincinnati, Ohio, United States of America
[2]Cincinnati Children's Hospital Medical Center, Department of Infectious Disease, Cincinnati, Ohio, United States of America
[3]Cincinnati Children's Hospital Medical Center, Department of Biostatistics and Epidemiology, Cincinnati, Ohio, United States of America
[4]Centers for Disease Control and Prevention, Division of Viral Diseases, Atlanta, Georgia, United States of America
[5]University of Cincinnati College of Allied Health Sciences, Department of Rehabilitation, Exercise and Nutrition Science, Cincinnati, Ohio, United States of America
[6]Cherokee Nation Assurance, Arlington, Virginia, United States of America
[7]Centers for Disease Control and Prevention, Division of Foodborne, Waterborne, and Environmental Diseases, Atlanta, Georgia, United States of America

---

[*] *Correspondence:* Ardythe Morrow, PhD, University of Cincinnati College of Medicine, Department of Environmental and Public Health, 160 Panzeca Way, Cincinnati, OH 45202, United States. Email: morrowa@ucmail.uc.edu.

In: Environmental Health
Editors: I Leslie Rubin and Joav Merrick
ISBN: 979-8-88697-292-4

Abstract

Nearly 14% of American children aged 2–5 have obesity, with higher rates in children from lower-income and Black families. While evidence connects neighborhood socio-economic environment (SEE) and obesity in adults and adolescents, little is known of this relationship in young children. We compared measures of SEE and family-level socio-demographic factors as predictors of obesity at age two. *Methods*: Family-level data from the PREVAIL Cohort, a CDC-funded birth cohort in Cincinnati, Ohio, were collected prenatally from the mothers. Residential addresses were geocoded and assigned validated measures of census tract-level SEE, including USDA food desert indicators and the Deprivation Index. Family-level and ecological SEE were compared as predictors of obesity (BMI*z* ≥1.65) at age two in terms of proportional differences, relative risk, and model fit statistics. *Results*: Residing outside of Deprivation Index High SEE neighborhoods was significantly associated with higher proportion (20.0% *vs* 5.9%; χ^2=4.36, *p*=0.037) and increased risk of obesity in univariable (RR = 3.4, 95%CI: 1.26–13.86) and multivariable models (RR = 3.5, 95%CI: 1.06–11.71). There were no differences in proportion or risk of obesity by USDA food desert indicators or family-level factors. Models using categorical Deprivation Index performed better than the family-level and the USDA food desert variables in terms of model fit. *Conclusion*: In the PREVAIL Cohort, only category of Deprivation Index was a significant predictor of obesity in two-year-old children. Future studies are needed to evaluate the Deprivation Index as a generalizable tool to identify neighborhoods at higher risk for obesity.

Introduction

Childhood obesity is a growing epidemic in the United States (US) and increases risks for a wide range of metabolic, vascular, and endocrine disorders throughout life (1, 2). Although children aged 12-19 years have the highest obesity rates in childhood (20.7%), nearly 14% of children 2 – 5 years of age meet obesity criteria, a rate that has more than doubled in the last five decades, with significant differences by income category, family education level, race, and ethnicity (3-5). This is especially important, as early childhood obesity is a strong predictor of obesity and obesity-related comorbidities in adolescence and adulthood and can contribute to health disparities in low income and minority populations throughout life (1, 2, 6).

Evidence shows that weight status and obesity in older children and adults is intimately connected to a network of social, structural, racial, and economic differences in family and neighborhood environments (7-12). While this relationship in younger children is understudied, factors that influence parent and sibling weight status are shown to affect the weight status of younger children in the household (13, 14) and socio-demographic measures associated with differences in child obesity risk are correlated with residential neighborhood (15, 16).

However, most studies in the US linking environmental indicators and childhood obesity have focused on the food access environment (i.e., food deserts) rather than socio-economic environment (SEE) and have reported inconsistent results. Two recent systematic reviews found that, while results were generally supportive of a connection between neighborhood food environments and child obesity, results were inconsistent (17, 18). Mei et al. (18) hypothesized that the inconsistency in findings could be due to contextual factors such as individual family characteristics, including race, income, and education; Cobb et al. (17) identified a differential effect between food access and obesity when stratifying children by aggregate neighborhood income, suggesting that food access alone is not a sufficient measure of neighborhood environment.

A validated, national source of ecological socio-economic and food access data is the US Census Bureau's annual American Community Survey (ACS) (19). The ACS includes detailed questions regarding social and economic status in a representative annual sample of US residents, such as education level, use of social services, family income, and vehicle ownership. Data are compiled by US census tract, which is generally aligned with neighborhoods in urban environments, and has been used to create two validated sources of census tract-level measures of SEE, the USDA Food Access Research Atlas (formerly the Food Desert Locator) (20) and the Deprivation Index (21).

The Food Access Research Atlas contains multiple measures of food and socio-economic environment, including several binary indicators of census tract fresh food access and availability. Food Access Research Atlas variables are used widely to designate food deserts and have been correlated to higher rates of obesity in adults and school-aged children (22, 23). However, these binary variables have been inconsistently associated with earlier childhood obesity, may not fully reflect community socio-economic environment, and have been shown to more accurately reflect issues of access in rural than in urban neighborhoods (18, 24-28).

The Deprivation Index is a more granular measure of SEE that standardizes census tract aggregate material deprivation (19, 21). Although similar material deprivation indices have been shown to predict child weight status in other Western countries (29), and differences in other child health outcomes have been found by Deprivation Index score (21, 30, 31), the Deprivation Index has not, to our knowledge, been used in studies of childhood obesity in the US.

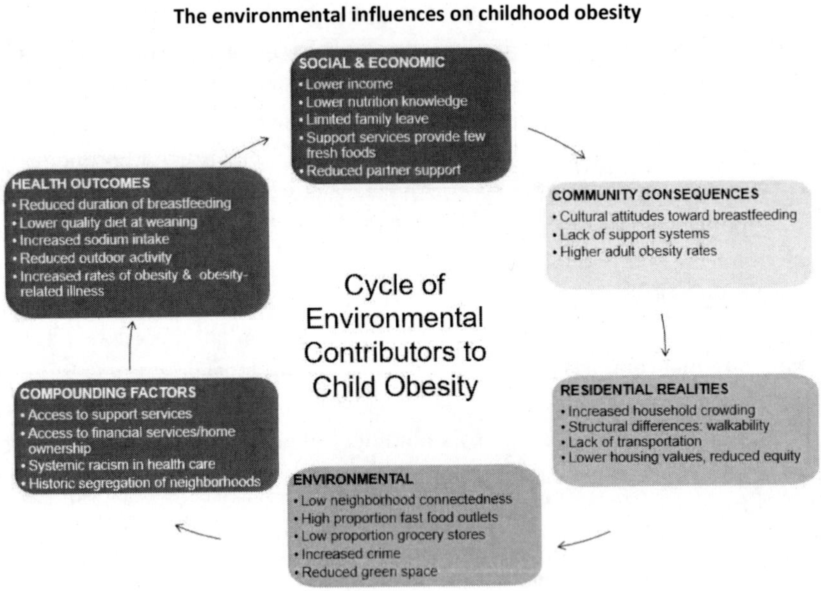

Figure 1. Childhood obesity is intimately linked to social, racial and economic differences in neighborhood environments (12). These differences contribute in myriad ways to a cycle of obesity and obesity-related comorbidities in low income and minority populations. While evidence of food access as a contributor to early childhood obesity has been mixed (17, 18) environmental factors, such as green space, neighborhood safety, and access to health care, are shown to predict obesity status in older children and adults (7, 8), while individual factors, such as race and income, are associated with both one's residential neighborhood and obesity risk (11, 15).

Here, we apply these validated measures of fresh food access and neighborhood material deprivation compared with individual family-level factors as potential predictors of risk of early childhood obesity. While both of these indices have been used previously to quantify neighborhood environment, validating USDA and Deprivation Index measures as predictors for obesity in young children could provide a powerful tool to guide public health initiatives by identifying regions of early disparities in weight status, potentially breaking the cycle of obesity and obesity-related health disparities in low-income and minority populations (see Figure 1).

Our study

The Pediatric Respiratory and Enteric Virus Acquisition and Immunogenesis Longitudinal Cohort (PREVAIL), a prospective two-year birth cohort study in Cincinnati, Ohio, was approved by the Institutional Review Boards at the US Centers for Disease Control and Prevention (CDC) and Cincinnati Children's Hospital Medical Center. Participant enrollment began in April of 2017, and data collection was completed in October 2020. Study methods, including recruitment, enrollment, and data collection have previously been described (32); methods relevant to this work are described here. Inclusion criteria for the study were maternal age ≥18 years and delivery of a healthy, live-born, singleton infant at one of two urban study hospitals. Exclusion criteria included living more than 20 miles from the birth hospital, illicit drug use, major congenital anomaly in the infant, gestational age under 35 weeks, or HIV infection. Provisional enrollment occurred in the third trimester of pregnancy, and final eligibility and study enrollment was determined at a two-week post-partum home visit. Mother-infant dyads were followed from birth until age two through weekly text surveillance and periodic in-clinic study visits. This analysis is a subset of the PREVAIL Cohort, including only those subjects who completed the end-of-study (month 24) visit.

Family-level data

Family-level socio-demographic data were collected in-person at baseline (third trimester of pregnancy). Maternal race was categorized as White, Black, or other (biracial, Asian, Native American, Pacific Islander, or unknown). Due to the small number of participants who identified as Hispanic (<5%), ethnicity was not included as a covariate in this analysis; subjects who identified as ethnically Hispanic were included in their self-identified racial group. Maternal education level was defined as completion of any post-secondary education or training (>HS) or less (≤HS). Maternal marital status was defined as married or not, independent of cohabitation status, while living with a partner was defined as cohabitation with a significant other, independent of marital status. Insurance status was categorized as public or private, with the few families who were uninsured orqualifying for both public and private insurance classified as publicly insured. Family income level was grouped in line with the Federal Poverty Level for a family of four (<$25,000/year), between 100% and 200% of Federal Poverty Level ($25,000-$50,000/year) and above (>$50,000/year). Maternal age was calculated based on the mother's age at the time of the child's birth.

Maternal weight and height from the first trimester of pregnancy were abstracted from the obstetrics medical record for nearly all (94.7%) mothers. When this time point was not available, the maternal-recalled height and pre-pregnancy weight was used. Maternal BMI was calculated as kg/m^2 and presence of obesity was defined as a BMI of >30 (33). Sensitivity analysis found no significant differences when excluding mothers with recalled weight and height from analysis.

Neighborhood data

Family residential address was reported at the baseline visit and updated, if changed, in REDCap data management software (34). All PREVAIL subject addresses were geocoded to the census tract-level using DeGAUSS software (35). Residential addresses reported at the month 24 visit were used for all analyses. To quantify neighborhood fresh food access, we assigned corresponding 2015 USDA Food Access Research Atlas variables: Low Income (a high percentage of the population at or below the federal poverty level or median income of the region), Low Access (≥100 residents of the tract live more than one-half mile (urban) or 10 miles (rural) from a grocery store and do not own a vehicle) and Low Income/Low Access (LILA, census tracts that meet both Low Income and Low Access criteria) (20).

To quantify neighborhood material deprivation, we assigned Deprivation Index scores (21). The Deprivation Index combines six ACS census tract-level variables: 1) percentage of vacant homes, 2) median home value; and the percentage of the population who 3) are without a high school diploma, 4) have used any government social-services or income support within 12 months, 5) lack health insurance, and 6) meet the federal definition of poverty, using a principal components analysis (19, 21). The score was then standardized into a continuous variable between 0 and 1, with increasing score representing increasing neighborhood deprivation (21).

Deprivation Index category was calculated by first averaging each family's Deprivation Index scores from all visits, then calculating quartiles of scores from the averages. Census tracts were grouped by quartile of score into High SEE (least deprived quartile), High-Mid and Low-Mid (intermediate quartiles) and Low SEE (most deprived quartile). As children in middle- and low-income families have been shown to have significantly different obesity rates than those in the highest income bracket (5), a binary variable indicating residence in the High SEE quartile or the remaining cohort (Not High SEE) was also assessed. A map of Deprivation Index and LILA census tracts included in this analysis can be found in Figure 2.

Maps of the PREVAIL Cohort catchment area categorized by measures of census tract socio-economic environment

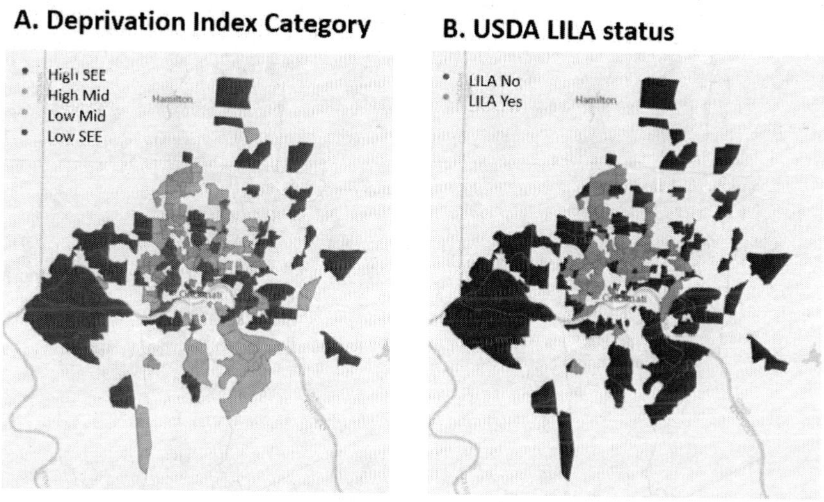

Figure 2. Maps of census tracts included in the PREVAIL Cohort, a CDC-funded birth cohort in Cincinnati, OH, color-coded by Deprivation Index Category (A) and USDA Low Income/Low Access (LILA, B) status. Residential addresses were geocoded to the census tract level and assigned Deprivation Index (21) and USDA Food Access Research Atlas (20) indicators of socio-economic environment (SEE). Deprivation Index category was assigned based on quartile of score, with the lowest quartile of scores indicating the least deprived census tracts (High SEE) and highest quartile of scores designated as the most deprived census tracts (Low SEE). LILA designation was used to identify census tracts that met both USDA Low Income and Low Access criteria, a frequently used food desert indicator.

Child obesity status

Age and sex normative body mass index *z* scores (BMI*z*) from the 24 month study visit were calculated using the parameters provided by the CDC National Center for Health Statistics (36). Presence of obesity was defined as a BMIz score ≥1.65 at age two (37). Imputation for erroneous entries (<0.5% of all entries) was performed by averaging the BMI*z* score from the two proximal visits. Sensitivity analysis found no significant differences in obesity rates after removing these imputations.

Statistical analysis

Power was calculated post-hoc, based on the number that completed the month 24 study visit. All analytic methods had at least 80% power to detect a minimum of 1.75-fold increase in obesity risk at a significance level of 0.05.

Fisher's exact test was used to identify differences in proportions for categorical and Kruskal-Wallis identified differences in medians of continuous family-level factors by SEE categories. Spearman correlations were calculated between each family socio-demographic factor and neighborhood SEE indicator. Differences in obesity proportions were tested using a Pearson χ^2 test with Yates continuity corrections. Log binomial regression assessed risk of obesity at 24 months of age, first in univariable models with each measure, then as multivariable models with Deprivation Index score, category, or LILA designation and family measures that met non-multi-collinearity criteria and produced converged models. Model fit was assessed by comparing each model's Akaike Information Criteria (AIC), the percent of variance explained by the model (R^2), and the Area Under the Receiver Operator Characteristic Curve (AUROC), with higher AUROC and R^2 and lower AIC associated with better model fit and an AUROC ≥ 0.70 considered adequate predictive value. Models were compared to each other using DeLong's test for correlated AUROC, with a significant test indicating a significant difference in predictive accuracy between models.

Comparisons were made with the highest SEE category as the reference group unless otherwise specified. The continuous Deprivation Index score was base 10 log-transformed for all analyses. Results are reported as estimate and 95% confidence interval, except where indicated. All analysis was performed using the R Environment for Statistical Computing (38).

Our findings

PREVAIL enrolled a total of 245 participants, of which 171 (69.8%) completed the month 24 visit and were included in this analysis (see Table 1). The cohort was racially and economically diverse, with 40.9% of mothers self-reporting as Black, 45.0% reporting incomes at or below $50,000 per year, and public and private insurance status equally distributed. Only six subjects (2.4%) identified as Hispanic ethnicity; three identified their race as Black, two as other, and one as White. Over one-third of the mothers (38.6%) completed no post-secondary training or education. Over half (57.3%) were married, while 70.1% reported living with a partner. The overall rate of maternal obesity (41.5%) was modestly higher than the NHANES-reported obesity rates for female adult (20-39 years) in the US (39.7%) (33).

Significant differences were found by SEE in the proportion of all family-level demographic factors, with increasing material deprivation, USDA Low Income, and LILA designations corresponding with increasing proportion of Black race, public insurance, unmarried status, lower maternal education, and lower income level (Table 1, all $p<0.01$). The proportion of mothers with obesity differed only by Low Income status ($p=0.030$).

Correlations were moderate to high between all family-level factors and Deprivation Index score, category, Low Income, and LILA (see Table 2). Low Access designation, however, was only modestly associated with family socio-demographic factors, and negatively associated with the lower socio-demographic category. For example, residence in Low Access census tracts was negatively correlated to unmarried status, lower education level, Deprivation Index score and category, and income <$25,000/year (all $p<0.05$).

Overall, 15.8% of the children in the cohort had obesity (27/171). Proportion of obesity significantly differed by SEE only in comparing the binary Deprivation Index High SEE (3/51, 5.9%) to the remaining cohort (24/120, 20.0%; $\chi^2=4.36$, $p=0.037$). In univariable log binomial models (see Table 3), only High Mid (RR 3.48 (95%CI: 1.12, 14.97)) and Low Mid (RR 3.40 (95%CI: 1.06, 14.79)) in the Deprivation Index categorical model and Not High SEE (RR 3.40 (95%CI: 1.26-13.86)) in the binary model were associated with significant increases in obesity risk. In terms of model fit, both categorical and binary Deprivation Index explained the highest percentage of variance (Table 3, $R^2=0.062$), and the binary Not High SEE model had the second-lowest AIC (Table 3, 146.92). However, none of the models met adequate prediction criteria (all AUROC <0.70), and none of the AUROC significantly differed per DeLong's test.

Table 1. Family-level socio-demographics of the PREVAIL Cohort by measures of neighborhood socio-economic environment

			DEPRIVATION INDEX CATEGORIES					*USDA FOOD ACCESS RESEARCH ATLAS CATEGORIES*					
		Total	**High SEE**	**High Mid SEE**	**Low Mid SEE**	**Low SEE**	***p***	***Low Income***	***p***	***Low Access***	***p***	***LILA***	***p***
		171	51 (29.8%)	44 (25.7%)	40 (23.4%)	36 (21.1%)		86 (50.3%)		153 (89.5%)		71 (41.5%)	
RACE	Black	70 (40.9%)	6 (11.8%)	14 (31.8%)	19 (47.5%)	31 (86.1%)	<0.001	57 (66.3%)	<0.001	60 (39.2%)	0.308	47 (66.2%)	<0.001
	White	94 (55.0%)	44 (86.3%)	28 (63.6%)	18 (45.0%)	4 (11.1%)		25 (29.1%)		87 (56.9%)		20 (28.2%)	
	Other	7 (4.1%)	1 (2.0%)	2 (4.6%)	3 (7.5%)	1 (2.8%)		4 (4.7%)		6 (3.9%)		4 (5.6%)	
INCOME LEVEL	<$25,000/yr	45 (26.3%)	4 (7.8%)	6 (13.6%)	13 (32.5%)	22 (61.1%)	<0.001	37 (43.0%)	<0.001	36 (23.5%)	0.045	28 (39.4%)	<0.001
	$25-50,000/yr	32 (18.7%)	3 (5.9%)	6 (13.6%)	14 (35.0%)	9 (25.0%)		25 (29.1%)		31 (20.3%)		24 (33.8%)	
	>$50,000/yr	94 (55.0%)	44 (86.3%)	32 (72.8%)	13 (32.5%)	5 (13.9%)		24 (27.9%)		86 (56.2%)		19 (26.8%)	
INSURANCE	Public	85 (49.7%)	10 (19.6%)	15 (34.1%)	27 (67.5%)	33 (91.7%)	<0.001	66 (76.7%)	<0.001	72 (47.1%)	0.049	54 (76.1%)	<0.001
	Private	86 (50.3%)	41 (80.4%)	29 (65.9%)	13 (32.5%)	3 (8.3%)		20 (23.3%)		81 (52.9%)		17 (23.9%)	
MATERNAL EDUC	≤High School	66 (38.6%)	5 (9.8%)	12 (27.3%)	18 (45.0%)	31 (86.1%)	<0.001	52 (62.5%)	<0.001	55 (35.9%)	0.044	41 (57.7%)	<0.001
	>High School	105 (61.4%)	46 (90.2%)	32 (72.7%)	22 (55.0%)	5 (13.9%)		34 (37.5%)		98 (64.1%)		30 (42.3%)	
MARITAL STATUS	Unmarried	73 (42.7%)	8 (15.7%)	12 (27.3%)	24 (60.0%)	29 (80.6%)	<0.001	56 (65.1%)	<0.001	60 (39.2%)	0.011	44 (62.0%)	<0.001
	Married	98 (57.3%)	43 (84.3%)	32 (72.7%)	16 (40.0%	7 (19.4%)		30 (34.9%)		93 (60.7%)		27 (38.0%)	
LIVES WITH PARTNER*	No	50 (29.9%)	6 (12.0%)	8 (18.6%)	14 (35.0%)	22 (64.7%)	<0.001	38 (45.8%)	<0.001	41 (27.5%)	0.059	29 (42.6%)	0.003
	Yes	117 (70.1%)	44 (88.0%)	35 (81.4%)	26 (65.0%)	12 (35.3%)		45 (54.2%)		108 (72.5%)		39 (57.4%)	
MATERNAL OBESITY**	No	100 (58.5%)	33 (64.7%)	27 (61.4%)	23 (57.5%)	17 (47.2%)	0.420	43 (50.0%)	0.030	92 (60.1%)	0.216	37 (52.1%)	0.161
	Yes	71 (41.5%)	18 (35.3%)	17 (38.6%)	13 (42.5%)	19 (52.8%)		43 (50.0%)		61 (39.9%)		34 (47.9%)	

Demographic distribution by measures of neighborhood socio-economic environment (SEE) in the PREVAIL Cohort (n=171). Residential addresses were geocoded and assigned validated measures of census tract-level SEE, including the Deprivation Index and USDA low income and low access variables. Categorical Deprivation Index was based on quartile of score (High, High Mid, Low Mid, and Low SEE) and a low income/low access (LILA) designation was defined as census tracts that met both USDA low income and low access criteria. Comparisons were made using Fisher's Exact test, with a significant p-value indicating that the proportionate distribution of each factor differed by SEE category.

*Cohabitation data was missing for n=4 subjects.

**Maternal obesity was calculated based on the height and weight reported in the obstetrics record from the first trimester of pregnancy and defined as $kg/m^2 \geq 30$.

Table 2. Correlations between neighborhood socio-economic environment and family-level measures in the PREVAIL Cohort

	Black Race	Maternal Age	Lower Income Level	Public Insurance	Lower Maternal Educ	Married	Lives with Partner	Dep. Index Score	Dep. Index Category	LILA	Low Income	Low Access
Black Race		-0.30	0.66	0.77	0.63	-0.58	-0.63	0.56	0.53	0.43	0.52	-0.10
Maternal Age	<0.001		-0.31	-0.35	-0.43	0.31	0.24	-0.28	-0.31	-0.20	-0.20	-0.04
Lower Income Level	<0.001	<0.001		0.81	0.71	-0.72	-0.63	0.60	0.57	0.43	0.53	-0.12
Public Insurance	<0.001	<0.001	<0.001		0.70	-0.75	-0.63	0.58	0.55	0.44	0.54	-0.15
Lower Maternal Educ	<0.001	<0.001	<0.001	<0.001		-0.60	-0.61	0.58	0.55	0.33	0.45	-0.16
Married	<0.001	<0.001	<0.001	<0.001	<0.001		0.65	-0.54	-0.50	-0.33	-0.46	0.20
Lives with Partner	<0.001	0.002	<0.001	<0.001	<0.001	<0.001		-0.43	-0.40	-0.23	-0.34	0.15
Deprivation Index Score	<0.001	<0.001	<0.001	<0.001	<0.001	<0.001	<0.001		0.97	0.62	0.82	-0.30
Deprivation Index Category	<0.001	<0.001	<0.001	<0.001	<0.001	<0.001	<0.001	<0.001		0.64	0.82	-0.26
LILA	<0.001	0.008	<0.001	<0.001	<0.001	<0.001	<0.001	<0.001	<0.001		0.84	0.29
Low Income	<0.001	0.007	<0.001	<0.001	<0.001	<0.001	<0.001	<0.001	<0.001	<0.001		-0.23
Low Access	0.184	0.645	0.113	0.044	0.038	0.007	0.050	<0.001	0.001	<0.001	0.003	

Spearman correlation coefficients (unshaded) and *p* values (shaded) for measures of neighborhood socio-economic environment (SEE) and family-level factors in the PREVAIL Cohort (*n*=171). Residential addresses were geocoded and assigned validated measures of census tract-level SEE, including the Deprivation Index and USDA low income and low access variables. Categorical Deprivation Index was based on quartile of score and a low income/low access (LILA) designation was defined as census tracts that met both USDA low income and low access criteria.

Table 3. Log binomial models for obesity risk at age two in the prevail cohort

	Variable	Level	RR	95%CI	R^2	AIC	AUROC
UNIVARIABLE MODELS	Deprivation Index score	Log10(score)	4.75	0.69 – 33.34	0.025	150.68	0.597
	Deprivation Index category	Low SEE [1]	3.31	0.99 – 14.57	0.062	150.90	0.615
		Low Mid [1]	3.40	1.06 – 14.79			
		High Mid [1]	3.48	1.12 – 14.97			
	Not High SEE	Yes [1]	3.40	1.26 – 13.86	0.062	146.92	0.611
	Low income	Yes [2]	1.68	0.83 – 3.61	0.021	151.09	0.575
	Low access [a, b]	Yes [3]	0.68	0.30 – 2.11	0.006	152.59	0.526
	LILA	Yes [4]	1.52	0.75 – 3.08	0.014	151.78	0.561
	Race	Black [5]	1.34	0.63 – 2.85	0.036	151.50	0.521
		Other [5]	3.36	0.93 – 8.07			
	Maternal Educ	≤High School [6]	1.09	0.52 – 2.19	0.001	153.11	0.513
	Maternal Age	Years	1.03	0.96 – 1.11	0.009	152.32	0.563
	Income Level	<$25k/year [7]	0.89	0.39 – 2.22	0.011	154.07	0.552
		$25-50k/year [7]	1.41	0.53 – 3.74			
	Insurance	Public [8]	1.26	0.63 – 2.60	0.004	152.73	0.535
	Marital status	Unmarried [9]	1.45	0.72 – 2.93	0.011	152.08	0.554
	Lives with Partner	No [10]	0.91	0.37 – 1.95	0.001	144.96	0.511
	Maternal obesity	Yes [11]	1.31	0.65 – 2.6	0.006	152.59	0.539

	Variable	Level	RR	95%CI	R^2	AIC	AUROC
MULTIVARIABLE MODELS	Deprivation Index Score	Log(10) score	8.29	0.65 – 108.48			
	+ race	Black [5]	1.14	0.38 – 3.18			
	+ maternal education	Other [5]	3.03	0.82 – 7.67	0.068	154.3	0.644
	+ maternal obesity	≤High School 1[6]	0.62	0.23 – 1.70			
		Mat. obesity [11]	1.24	0.59 – 2.60			
	Deprivation Index category	Low SEE [1]	3.88	0.90 – 16.73			
	+ race	Low Mid [1]	3.29	0.89 – 12.13			
	+ maternal education	High Mid [1]	3.63	1.04 – 12.68			
	+ maternal obesity [a]	Black [5]	1.19	0.44 – 3.17	0.099	155.1	0.674
		Other [5]	2.93	1.08 – 7.93			
		≤High School [6]	0.65	0.26 – 1.64			
		Mat. obesity [11]	1.19	0.58 – 2.45			
	Not High SEE	Yes [1]	3.52	1.06 – 11.71	0.098	151.1	0.674
	+ race	Black [5]	1.17	0.44 – 3.09			
	+ maternal education	Other [5]	2.81	1.06 – 7.49			
	+ maternal obesity [b]	≤High School [6]	0.69	0.29 – 1.64			
		Mat. obesity [11]	1.18	0.58 – 2.41			
	LILA	Yes [4]	1.36	0.63 – 2.97	0.048	156.3	0.613
	+ race	Black [5]	1.24	0.40 – 3.50			
	+ maternal education	Other [5]	3.10	0.83 – 8.04			
	+ maternal obesity	≤High School 1[6]	0.84	0.34 – 2.13			
		Mat. obesity [11]	1.20	0.57 – 2.52			

Log binomial models of risk of obesity at age two for children enrolled in the PREVAIL cohort (n=171) by family-level socio-demographic and neighborhood socio-economic environment (SEE). Residential addresses were geocoded and assigned validated measures of census tract-level SEE, including the Deprivation Index and USDA low income and low access variables. Categorical Deprivation Index was based on quartile of score and a low income/low access (LILA) designation was defined as census tracts that met both USDA low income and low access criteria. An area under the receiver operator characteristic curve (AUROC) ≥0.70 was considered adequate predictive accuracy, with higher variance explained (R^2) and lower Akaike information criterion (AIC) indicating better model fit. Superscript letters indicate significant differences in AUROC per DeLong's test for correlated AUROC for the model comparisons.

Reference values are [1]High SEE, [2]not Low Income, [3]not Low Access, [4]not LILA, [5]white race, [6]> high school education level, [7]income > $50,000/year, [8]private insurance, [9]married, [10]cohabitating, [11]no maternal obesity.

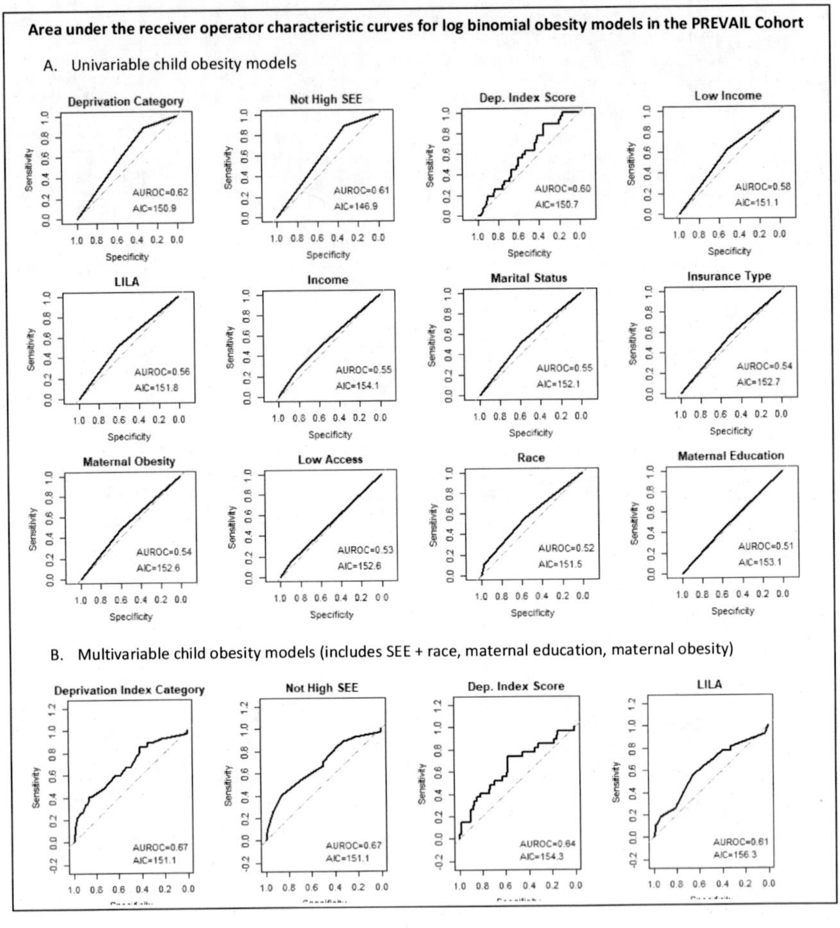

Figure 3. Visualizations of areas under the receiver characteristic curves (AUROC) for log binomial models of obesity risk in two-year-old children enrolled in the PREVAIL Cohort. Residential addresses were geocoded and assigned two validated measures of census tract socio-economic environment (SEE), the Deprivation Index (21) and the USDA Food Access Research Atlas variables Low Income, Low Access, and Low Income/Low Access (LILA) (20). Deprivation Index categories were assigned based on quartile of Deprivation Index score. A binary comparison of the Least Deprived quartile compared to the remaining cohort was also included. Family-level factors were collected at the baseline study visit from the mother. Univariable models assessed risk of obesity at age two by each variable. Multivariable models included measures of SEE and the family-level variables of maternal race, education level, and presence of obesity. Model fit was compared for univariable (A) and multivariable (B) models using Akaike Information criteria (AIC) and area under the receiver operator characteristic curve (AUROC), with lower AIC and higher AUROC indicating better model fit, and an AUROC $\geq$0.70 considered adequate predictive accuracy.

Due to issues of model convergence, multivariable log binomial models were limited to the SEE variables of Deprivation Index score, Deprivation Index category, Not High SEE, and LILA, and the family-level variables of race, maternal education level, and maternal obesity. Increased risk of child obesity was associated with residence in High Mid (RR 3.63 (95%CI 1.04–12.68)) in the categorical Deprivation Index model and residing outside of the High SEE census tracts (RR 3.52 (95%CI 1.06–11.71) in the binary Deprivation Index model. In terms of model fit, multivariable models using the Deprivation Index, including the log(10) of Deprivation index score, category, and Not High SEE, had higher R^2 than any of the univariable models. In comparing all model AUROC (Figure 3, A & B), the Deprivation Index category and Not High SEE multivariable models had significantly greater AUROC than the univariable model for Low Access. No other model, whether univariable or multivariable, significantly differed in AUROC; no model explained over 10% of the variance, and none of the models met adequate prediction criteria (Figure 3, all AUROC < 0.70).

Discussion

In the PREVAIL Cohort, 15.8% of children had obesity at age two. Significant differences in the proportion of obesity at age two were identified only when comparing the Deprivation Index High SEE census tracts to the remaining cohort; we found no differences in obesity rates among individual Deprivation Index categories, any of the USDA Food Access Research Atlas variables, or any of the family-level socio-demographic factors. In regression models, residing in either of the Deprivation Index intermediate SEE categories or in any neighborhood outside of the High SEE neighborhoods was associated with ≥ 3.4 times the risk of obesity, a relationship that did not significantly change when controlling for subject race, maternal education level, and presence of maternal obesity. When analyzing obesity risk in relation to the binary USDA Low Income, Low Access, or LILA designations, no differences were identified. When comparing model performance, all univariable and multivariable models were similar in model fit, and there were few differences in terms of predictive accuracy. Despite significant associations with obesity risk, none of the models met criteria for adequate model prediction and none explained more than 10% of the variance.

Previous studies using NHANES data have identified family-level socio-demographic indicators as risk factors for increased obesity in children as young as two years (3, 4). None of our family-level variables were significant in univariable or multivariable analysis of obesity risk, and no differences in obesity proportions were identified by any of these factors. However, we did find moderate to high correlations between all of these factors and our ecological measures of SEE and significant differences in the proportional distribution of family demographic factors by most SEE measures. Further examination of the distribution by Deprivation Index category found that these differences were mostly between the High SEE group and the remaining cohort. The High SEE group was 11.8% Black, 7.8% reported a family income below $25,000/year, and 91.2% had completed at least 2 years of post-secondary education or training. The remaining cohort, in contrast, was 53.3% Black, 34.2% were at the lowest income level, and 49.2% were in the higher education category (all $p<0.001$). Importantly, these differences align with family-level factors previously associated with child obesity risk (3, 4, 37).

That obesity differences were found using the Deprivation Index to categorize neighborhood SEE and not by the more commonly used USDA food desert variables in our study is unsurprising, given the inconsistency of findings surrounding child obesity and food deserts (17, 18). The Deprivation Index's inclusion of aggregated socio-demographic variables, such as education level and use of public assistance, provides more granularity compared to the binary USDA measures, and includes variables shown on an individual level to be associated with increased obesity. This was especially true with the frequently used Low Access variable, which had the lowest R^2 and AUROC and the highest AIC of all of the ecological univariable models and was the only model to have a significantly lower AUROC compared to any other model. While not significantly different in terms of predictive value from the Deprivation Index models, the models including Low Income and LILA also failed to find significant risk of obesity in our population and had inferior model fit statistics compared to all permutations of the Deprivation Index. The lack of significance in the USDA measures as predictors of child obesity suggests that the associations between neighborhood SEE and child weight are more complex than simply neighborhood average income level or access to a grocery store.

That neighborhoods can be best categorized by multiple indicators of material deprivation is illustrative of the socio-demographic segregation found at either end of the affluence spectrum in the U.S. While lending policies of the early to mid-20th century resulted in the segregation of Black Americans into increasingly impoverished urban centers, higher-income, White residents moved from the urban core into newer, wealthier exurbs and suburbs (16). We detected this pattern in Deprivation Index and LILA maps of PREVAIL census tracts (see Figure 2). Clear clustering of increasing neighborhood deprivation is seen in the urban center, with lower deprivation radiating to the exurban and suburban areas.

In 1993, Massey and Denton found that race and neighborhood were so collinear as to make it "impossible to precisely estimate their separate effects" (16). More recent studies, however, have found that multiplicative levels of segregation, including inter- and intra-racial income segregation, can be used to examine health disparities including obesity (11, 15, 39). This segregation, along lines associated with obesity risk, explains why differences in these factors are significantly different by neighborhood SEE and why the more granular Deprivation Index outperforms the binary USDA variables.

Consistent with the above, we found a high level of racial and income segregation, with low-income Black mothers over five times as likely to live in the Low SEE neighborhoods than low-income White mothers. We also found that adding additional socio-demographic variables, outside of race and maternal education, to our neighborhood models of obesity risk resulted in a failure in our models to converge, suggesting an overfitting of the models, possibly due to insufficient sample size and high multicollinearity between our subjects' family demographics and neighborhood of residence.

Limitations

Our analysis has some limitations. Domestic stressors, such as neighborhood crime, financial hardship and food security, as well as structural elements, such as green space and walkability, have been significantly associated with increased risk of obesity in older children (7, 8, 40, 41). We did not account for these factors, and the only structural variable that we included, Low Access, was found to have limited validity in this context. However, given the strong association with individual family-level factors and neighborhood SEE, the possibility that these other measures of neighborhood environment contributed to our outcomes cannot be discounted. As we were primarily interested in comparing the predictive power of our measures, testing the multiplicative effects of segregation was outside of the scope of this project. Future work should include measures of segregation, and interaction by race or education level, which may better clarify causality and improve the models' predictive value. While ethnicity has been shown to be a risk factor for childhood obesity (3), due to limited numbers of subjects who identified as

Hispanic (n=6, 2.4%), we were unable to include ethnicity in our analysis. However, our population was representative of Cincinnati and the birth hospitals from which we recruited (32). Future studies are needed with larger, more geographically and ethnically diverse, populations.

Finally, these data were drawn only from the last visit (month 24) of a birth cohort, while allocation of Deprivation Index categories was based on quartiles of score at each study point from birth to age two. We did find significant differences in those lost-to-follow up (n=74) compared to those who completed the study at two years (n=171). Those lost-to-follow up were more likely to be publicly insured, in the lowest income group, younger, unmarried, and in the lower education group (all $p<0.01$). Of the ecological predictors, those lost to follow up lived in more deprived neighborhoods when comparing median Deprivation Index scores ($p=0.015$).

This differential drop-out may, in part, explain our finding that High SEE census tracts had decreased risk of obesity compared to the remaining cohort rather than when comparing across categories. Sensitivity analysis did not find any significant differences when allocating categories based on the 24-month visit alone and there was no significant difference in terms of obesity prevalence in those lost to follow up compared to those included in this analysis. However, the differential change in sample size, rather than a lack of effect, may have limited detection of differences in the Low SEE group in the categorical model, as evidenced by the similarity in effect sizes for the three categories outside of High SEE, and no significant difference in risk was found among the High Mid, Low Mid, and Low SEE categories.

Thus, given the correlations between Deprivation Index category and socio-demographic factors and the lack of significant differences in predictive value from both family-level demographics and USDA food desert indicators, we conclude that level of neighborhood deprivation, measured by the Deprivation Index, functions as a summary of multiple measures of family socio-demographic and economic factors and may be useful to identify neighborhoods at higher risk for early childhood obesity - a critical first step to breaking the cycle of obesity and obesity-related health disparities attributable to neighborhood environment. However, due to the small sample size, geographic restriction, and low ethnic diversity of this study population, further research is needed to consider neighborhood material deprivation, as measured by the Deprivation Index, a generalizable risk factor for child obesity in the US.

Conclusion

While it has been inconsistently shown that factors associated with the built environment such as food desert status, walkability, and recreational space, are associated with increased rates of childhood obesity, our approach showed that areas of increased obesity risk can be identified by examining a more granular measure of SEE of the neighborhood, which is best summarized by the neighborhood's level of deprivation. We found that the Deprivation Index efficiently identified areas of increased risk of obesity in very young children in our population and appeared to perform better or on par with more commonly used measures, such as USDA food desert status and family-level socio-demographic factors. Future studies including more geographic and ethnic diversity and larger sample size are needed to validate this measure as a generalizable predictor of child obesity.

Acknowledgments

We gratefully acknowledge the participation of the PREVAIL birth cohort families. The authors also wish to thank our researchers at the University of Cincinnati, Cincinnati Children's Hospital, and The Christ Hospital – Cincinnati and gratefully acknowledge the hard work of the dedicated PREVAIL staff. This work was funded by a cooperative agreement from the US Centers for Disease Control and Prevention (IP16-004). Dr. Conrey received support from the Molecular Epidemiology in Children's Environmental Health Training program (grant 5 T32 ES 10957-18). Data management support was provided through the Center for Clinical and Translational Science and Training at the University of Cincinnati and Cincinnati Children's Hospital Medical Center (grant 2UL2TROO1425-05A1). Guidance, mentorship, and editorial assistance was provided by the Break the Cycle of Children's Environmental Health Disparities training program, based at Emory University in Atlanta, GA. The findings and conclusions in this report are those of the authors and do not necessarily represent the official position of the U.S. Centers for Disease Control and Prevention.

References

[1] Kelsey MM, Zaepfel A, Bjornstad P, Nadeau KJ. Age-related consequences of childhood obesity. Gerontology 2014;60(3):222-8.

[2] Llewellyn A, Simmonds M, Owen CG, Woolacott N. Childhood obesity as a predictor of morbidity in adulthood: a systematic review and meta-analysis. Obes Rev 2016;17(1):56-67.

[3] Ogden C, Fryar C, Martin C, Freedman D, Carroll M, Gu Q, et al. Trends in obesity prevalence by race and Hispanic origin—1999–2000 to 2017–2018. JAMA 2020;324(12):1208-10.

[4] Hales C, Carroll M, Fryar C, Ogden C. Prevalence of obesity and severe obesity among adults: United States, 2017–2018. NCHS Data Brief. Hyattsville, MD: National Center for Health Statistics, 2020:360.

[5] Ogden C, Carroll M, Fakhouri T, Hales C, Fryar C, Li X, et al. Prevalence of obesity among youths by household income and education level of head of household — United States 2011–2014. MMWR 2018;67:186-9.

[6] Vargas CM, Stines EM, Granado HS. Health-equity issues related to childhood obesity: a scoping review. J Public Health Dent 2017;77(S1):S32-42.

[7] Duncan DT, Sharifi M, Melly SJ, Marshall R, Sequist TD, Rifas-Shiman SL, et al. Characteristics of walkable built environments and BMI z-scores in children: evidence from a large electronic health record database. Environ Health Perspect 2014;122(12):1359-65.

[8] Carroll-Scott A, Gilstad-Hayden K, Rosenthal L, Peters SM, McCaslin C, Joyce R, et al. Disentangling neighborhood contextual associations with child body mass index, diet, and physical activity: the role of built, socioeconomic, and social environments. Soc Sci Med 2013;95:106-14.

[9] Johnson KA, Showell NN, Flessa S, Janssen M, Reid N, Cheskin LJ, et al. Do neighborhoods matter? A systematic review of modifiable risk factors for obesity among low socio-economic status Black and Hispanic children. Child Obes 2019;15(2):71-86.

[10] Fiechtner L, Sharifi M, Sequist T, Block J, Duncan DT, Melly SJ, et al. Food environments and childhood weight status: effects of neighborhood median income. Child Obes 2015;11(3):260.

[11] Do DP, Frank R, Iceland J. Black-white metropolitan segregation and self-rated health: Investigating the role of neighborhood poverty. Soc Sci Med 2017;187:85-92.

[12] Davison KK, Birch LL. Childhood overweight: A contextual model and recommendations for future research. Obes Rev 2001;2(3):159-71.

[13] Saelens BE, Sallis JF, Frank LD, Couch SC, Zhou C, Colburn T, et al. Obesogenic neighborhood environments, child and parent obesity: The Neighborhood Impact on Kids study. Am J Prev Med 2012;42(5):e57.

[14] Kang Sim DE, Strong DR, Manzano MA, Rhee KE, Boutelle KN. Evaluation of dyadic changes of parent-child weight loss patterns during a family-based behavioral treatment for obesity. Pediatr Obes 2020;15(6):e12622.

[15] Quillian L. Segregation and poverty concentration: The role of three segregations. Am Sociol Rev 2012;77(3):354-79.

[16] Massey DS, Denton NA. American apartheid: segregation and the making of the underclass. Cambridge, MA: Harvard University Press,1993.

[17] Cobb LK, Appel LJ, Franco M, Jones-Smith JC, Nur A, Anderson CAM. The relationship of the local food environment with obesity: A systematic review of methods, study quality, and results. Obesity 2015;23(7):1331-44.

[18] Mei K, Huang H, Xia F, Hong A, Chen X, Zhang C, et al. State-of-the-art of measures of the obesogenic environment for children. Obes Rev 2020 Jul 28.

[19] American Community Survey. URL: https://www.census.gov/programs-surveys/acs.

[20] Food Access Research Atlas. URL: https://www.ers.usda.gov/data-products/food-access-research-atlas/.

[21] Brokamp C, Beck AF, Goyal NK, Ryan P, Greenberg JM, Hall ES. Material community deprivation and hospital utilization during the first year of life: an urban population–based cohort study. Ann Epidemiol 2019;30:37-43.

[22] Woodruff RC, Haardörfer R, Raskind IG, Hermstad A, Kegler MC. Comparing food desert residents with non-food desert residents on grocery shopping behaviours, diet and BMI: results from a propensity score analysis. Public Health Nutr 2020;23(5):806-11.

[23] Thomsen MR, Nayga RM, Alviola PA, Rouse HL. The effect of food deserts on the body mass index of elementary schoolchildren. Am J Agric Econ 2016;98(1):1-18.

[24] Briggs AC, Black AW, Lucas FL, Siewers AE, Fairfield KM. Association between the food and physical activity environment, obesity, and cardiovascular health across Maine counties. BMC Public Health 2019;19(1):374-9.

[25] MacNell L. A geo-ethnographic analysis of low-income rural and urban women's food shopping behaviors. Appetite 2018;128:311-20.

[26] Santorelli ML, Okeke JO. Evaluating community measures of healthy food access. J Commun Health 2017;42(5):991-7.

[27] Block JP, Subramanian SV. Moving beyond "food deserts": Reorienting United States policies to reduce disparities in diet quality. PLoS Med 2015;12(12):e1001914.

[28] Kimbro RT, Denney JT. Neighborhood context and racial/ethnic differences in young children's obesity: structural barriers to interventions. Soc Sci Med 2013;95:97.

[29] Phillips RL, Liaw W, Crampton P, Exeter DJ, Bazemore A, Vickery KD, et al. How other countries use deprivation indices-and why the United States desperately needs one. Health Aff (Millwood) 2016;35(11):1991-8.

[30] Brokamp C, Jandarov R, Rao MB, LeMasters G, Ryan P. Exposure assessment models for elemental components of particulate matter in an urban environment: A comparison of regression and random forest approaches. Atmos Environ 2017;151:1-11.

[31] Brokamp C, LeMasters GK, Ryan PH. Residential mobility impacts exposure assessment and community socioeconomic characteristics in longitudinal epidemiology studies. J Expo Sci Environ Epidemiol 2016;26(4):428-34.

[32] Morrow AL, Staat MA, DeFranco EA, McNeal MM, Cline AR, Conrey SC, et al. Pediatric respiratory and enteric virus acquisition and immunogenesis in US mothers and children aged 0-2: PREVAIL Cohort Study. JMIR Res Protoc 2021;12;10(2):e22222.

[33] Overweight and obesity. URL: https://www.cdc.gov/obesity/data/adult.html.

[34] Harris PA, Taylor R, Thielke R, Payne J, Gonzalez N, Conde JG. Research electronic data capture (REDCap) – A metadata-driven methodology and workflow process for providing translational research informatics support. J Biomed Inform 2009;42(2):377-81.

[35] Brokamp C. DeGAUSS: Decentralized Geomarker Assessment for Multi-Site Studies. J Open Source Software 2018;3(30):812.

[36] Growth charts-Z score data files. URL: https://www.cdc.gov/growthcharts/zscore.htm.

[37] Data, trend and maps. URL: https://www.cdc.gov/nccdphp/dnpao/data-trends-maps/index.html.

[38] R Core Team. R: A language and environment for statistical computing. Vienna, Austria: R Foundation for Statistical Computing, 2018. URL: https://www.R-project.org/.

[39] Anderson KF. Racial residential segregation and the distribution of health-related organizations in urban neighborhoods. Social Problems 2017;64(2):256-76.

[40] Metallinos-Katsaras, Elizabeth, PhD, RD, Must A, PhD, Gorman K, PhD. A longitudinal study of food insecurity on obesity in preschool children. J Acad Nutr Diet 2012;112(12):1949-58.

[41] Kim Y, Cubbin C, Oh S. A systematic review of neighbourhood economic context on child obesity and obesity-related behaviours. Obes Rev 2019;20(3):420-31.

Chapter 7

Investigating equitable access to greenspace during the COVID-19 pandemic: Implications for children's mental health in Durham, North Carolina

Sharmi Amin[*]**, Kate Hoffman, PhD, Catherine Kastleman, MPH and Heather M Stapleton, PhD**

Trinity College of Arts and Sciences, Duke University,
Durham and Nicholas School of the Environment, Duke University, Nicholas School of the Environment, Durham,
North Carolina, United States of America

Abstract

Past research suggests positive correlations between time spent outdoors and better mental health in children. During the COVID 19 pandemic, researchers predicted that limitations on social gathering could have lasting impacts on children's mental well-being. We hypothesized that protective guidelines set in place to prevent COVID-19 infection would decrease children's time spent in greenspaces, adversely impacting mental well-being. We also investigated changes in children's time spent outdoors during the pandemic, the social and structural barriers to accessing local greenspaces, and the potential impacts on children's mental health in Durham, North Carolina, USA. An online survey was distributed via parent Facebook groups to collect data (n = 95 children). The Pediatric Symptom Checklist (PSC) was used as a proxy for indicating children's mental well-being. Most parents indicated a change in the amount of time spent outside during the pandemic. Children who spent more time outdoors in general, and children who spent more time outdoors during the pandemic, had lower PSC scores, indicating better

[*] *Correspondence:* Email: sharmiamin@gmail.com.

mental well-being. When examining barriers to greenspace access, we observed no difference in the walkability index between higher- and lower-income zip codes. We did find that those residing in lower-income zip codes indicated more safety concerns about greenspaces particularly related to criminal activity. However, we found that the distribution of PSC scores was lower for children living in lower-income zip codes compared to higher-income zip codes, suggesting better mental well-being. Cumulatively, our results indicate that time spent outdoors has positive impacts on children's mental health.

Introduction

Greenspace is defined as space including grass, trees, or other vegetation that has been separated for recreational purposes within urban and suburban environments (1). A growing body of literature indicates that positive correlations exist between access to greenspace and greater mental well-being in children (2-5). Past studies have found that access to greenspace can have beneficial behavioral impacts on children, including improving attention, lessening health consequences of stress, and mitigating some symptoms of hyperactivity, in addition to overall improved physical and mental health outcomes (4, 5). More specifically, providing access to areas where children can interact with nature and peers has been suggested as an intervention to improve the mental well-being of children living in high-risk neighborhoods (4). However, access to greenspaces is often impacted by a community's socioeconomic status.

Elements such as sidewalks, traffic control, and physical proximity to greenspaces are generally more prevalent in higher-income neighborhoods (6). These factors not only improve perceptions of safety and security within these neighborhoods, but also have direct correlations with increased physical activity for children and overall health (5, 6). High-risk neighborhoods are often labelled as such due to a lack of these factors. These neighborhoods are characterized by patterns of social, economic, and environmental conditions that place residents "at-risk" of failure or of encountering obstacles in education, healthy lifestyles, employment, and self-sufficiency (7). Research has found that "walkability", a measure of how safe an urban environment is for pedestrians, in conjunction with perceived safety, play larger roles in the use of greenspaces than proximity (6). Thus, traffic risks, a lack of transportation, or no direct pathway are a few examples of patterns seen in high-risk neighborhoods that act as barriers that prevent children from being able to access or spend time outdoors safely (5). Recognizing that socioeconomic factors can impact the availability, accessibility, and use of greenspaces led us to consider factors such as walkability and potential safety concerns as we investigated changes in children's use of greenspace during the restrictive precautions at the early stages of the COVID-19 pandemic.

Considering the COVID-19 pandemic

Around March of 2020, the United States declared a public health emergency due to the SARS-CoV-2 (COVID-19) outbreak (8). In the following months, national and state governments issued stay-at-home or shelter-in-place orders and recommended a self-regulated quarantine for the public. Students across the nation were sent home from schools and education was rapidly transitioned to virtual platforms (9). With the onset of this unprecedented pandemic, early research suggested that this disruption of daily living patterns and dependence on virtual interaction could have lasting mental health consequences for children and adolescents due to reduced socialization and increased isolation indoors (9, 10). One study, which looked at changes in children's indoor/outdoor physical activity during the months of April-June 2020 found that a child's physical activity significantly declined after the onset of the restrictions imposed as a result of the pandemic (11). Since so much of children's physical activity is done in outdoor settings, and physical activity is recommended to ensure healthy development (11), we wanted to investigate how children's time spent outside changed as a result of the pandemic and associated external factors.

Data on changes in time spent outside over the course of the pandemic compared to pre-COVID-19 trends, and potential health impacts on children had not yet been analyzed in depth at the time of initiation of the study. Our goal was to collect data on these variables, identify barriers that limit children's access to greenspace, and explore potential correlations between access to greenspace and children's mental health as perceived by their parents. In this study, we compared how the amount of time children spend in greenspaces changed since the onset of the COVID-19 pandemic, the barriers that limit children's time spent outdoors, and implications for children's mental health in Durham, North Carolina, USA. We hypothesized that due to public health restrictions, children would spend less time outdoors during the COVID-19 pandemic, household income would be inversely associated with perceived barriers to greenspace access, and that greenspace utilization would be associated with higher perceived mental well-being in children as determined by their parent or guardian.

Our study

In January of 2021, we administered an online questionnaire to a convenience sample of parents regarding perceptions about access to greenspace and their children's outdoor activity before and during the pandemic. Recruitment for this study focused on Durham County in North Carolina, in the United States, where participants were introduced to the study and survey through Facebook Groups and participated via self-selection. The study and all protocols were reviewed and approved by the Duke University Institutional Review Board before initiation. To distribute the surveys, we requested access to 23 Facebook groups that came up in "Durham parents" or "Durham, NC" searches. We were given access to post the survey in 13 of these groups. Group sizes ranged from 60 to approximately 1,500 members, with groups categorized by faith, neighborhood, children's school system, etc. To participate in the study, individuals were required to live in a zip code within Durham County and have a child under the age of 18 years. All participating parents provided informed consent prior to completing the survey. The survey was posted two times in each group, with approximately one month between postings. The survey was closed after three months, at the end of March of 2021.

Parent questionnaires began with a brief demographic section, in which participants were asked about their child's race and ethnicity, and to choose their child's residential zip code from a drop-down menu of all Durham County zip codes. Part one of the survey asked questions regarding how the onset of the COVID-19 pandemic had changed children's time spent outside, using both qualitative and quantitative measures. Throughout the survey, "during the pandemic" was specified to describe the months of March through August of 2020. This time range was chosen to include some time in which families dealt with the transition from in-person to virtual school as well as a few of the following months that represented the height of the restrictions in response to the COVID-19 pandemic, up to the date of the survey. It should be noted that "time spent outdoors" and "time spent in [various types of] greenspaces" were used interchangeably to describe children spending time in outdoor settings. Part two of the survey asked questions about the walkability, safety, and accessibility of greenspaces within families' neighborhoods.

Finally, part three of the survey was a mental health survey completed by the parents using the Pediatric Symptom Checklist (PSC) (12). The PSC is a screening questionnaire used by health professionals to identify preliminary behavioral symptoms of psychosocial problems in children. It is scored on a continuous scale from 0-70, where lower scores indicate better mental well-being and higher scores indicate poorer mental well-being. Massachusetts General Hospital suggests that for children aged 5-16, a score of 28 or higher indicates that the child has more indicators of poor mental well-being than most other children within the age group and may benefit from further psychosocial functioning assessments (12). The PSC has been utilized previously as a mental health proxy when investigating sociological and environmental factors, in which children from economically disadvantaged care environments were significantly more likely to exhibit psychosocial impairment (13, 14).

Statistical analysis

We conducted a series of bivariate analyses using R-studio for select survey responses to examine associations between variables. We excluded any participants' data if Part 1 of the survey was not fully completed. For those that completed any question in Part 2, available data was used in analyses as long as participants provided responses for both variables being analyzed. As a consequence, the sample size used for each statistical analysis varied.

To evaluate associations between reported time spent outside and PSC score distributions, we used a Wilcoxon Signed Rank Test. Based on the survey and responses, the time spent outdoors was categorized into four intervals that included <1 hour, 1-3 hours, 3-4 hours, and >4 hours. A generalized linear model was used to identify significant differences between the average PSC scores for the different durations of time spent outside during the COVID-19 pandemic.

Based on the zip code selections in the demographic portion of the survey, our participants lived in nine different zip codes within Durham County. Zip codes were classified as either higher-income or lower-income (see table 1) using the median income of the zip codes included in the survey, (~$52,430) as a cut off point (15, 16). A Wilcoxon Signed Rank Test was used to assess differences in PSC score distributions between the higher-income and lower-income zip codes. A Chi-Squared Test was used to evaluate differences in the proportion of parents reporting concern for different safety factors between these higher- and lower-income zip codes.

Table 1. Participant demographic information

	Median Income	% Of Total Respondents (n = 95)	Demographic Distributions	Perceived Neighborhood Walkability		Average PSC Scores	Median PSC Score
				Walkable	Not Walkable		
Higher Income	$70, 973	74%	92% White 8% African American	61%	39%	23	22
Lower Income	$42, 563	26%	69% White 17% African American 6% Asian 6% American Indian	58%	42%	16	14

Our findings

One hundred twenty-one parents completed at least Part 1 of the survey. After excluding responses with incomplete data for other sections, 95 complete responses were used in the statistical analyses. All participants were residents of Durham County. Seventy of the 95 responses were from participants that reported living in higher-income zip codes, while 25 reported living in lower-income zip codes. In both higher-income and lower-income zip codes, respondents were predominately White (see Table 1). The demographic distributions of the higher and lower-income groups were not representative of the Durham County, which is approximately 49% White, 39% African American, 6% Asian, and 7% other races (17).

Changes in greenspace use

Ninety-one percent of total respondents reported that the amount of time that their children spent outside changed with the onset of the COVID-19 pandemic, and seventy percent indicated that their children's school transitioned to a completely virtual format during the months of March to June 2020. Before the onset of COVID, 30% of respondents indicated that the front or back yard of their home was where their child predominantly spent their time outdoors, with 70% indicating that their children predominantly used public greenspaces (i.e., neighborhood greenspaces, nearby parks or fields, schoolyard, or community playgrounds). After the onset of the pandemic, there was an increase in the number of respondents that indicated that a front or back yard was the primary greenspace used for recreation (65%) and a decrease in the number of participants reporting that their child predominantly used a public greenspace (35%). Parents were also asked to select concerns regarding access and use of their child's preferred greenspace. Of the respondents who selected risk of COVID-19 exposure as a safety concern (n = 47) within their child's preferred greenspace, 43% indicated that their child spent more time outside after the onset of the pandemic, but 57% reported that their children spent less time outside.

Children's mental health

To evaluate the potential implication of greenspace access and outdoor activity on children's mental health, we analyzed PSC scores in relation to time spent outside. In a previous study which used PSC scores to screen for psychosocial concerns for pediatric patients, Jellinek et al. (14) found that of 21,065 children, the average PSC score was 15.1. The average PSC score of the total respondent pool in this study was 23. Jellinek et al. (14) also found that overall prevalence rates of scores over 28, the cutoff for psychosocial dysfunction, were approximately 13% in school-aged children and 10% in pre-school aged children. While our study did not take age into account, 33% of the PSC scores reported for this study fell within the psychosocial dysfunction range. However, it is important to consider the impacts of the pandemic on reporting and children's PSC scores. The PSC includes information about time spent alone, school absences, and lowered interest in school; all factors which may have been impacted by restrictions on gathering and the transition to remote schooling. Jellinek et al. (14) found that children coming from low-income families were twice as likely to score within the range of psychosocial dysfunction (28-70) than those coming from higher-income families. Our study did not reflect this analysis; rather, the proportion of PSC scores within the psychosocial dysfunction range was higher in the higher-income group than lower-income group. There are many factors which may have contributed to these results, as discussed in later sections.

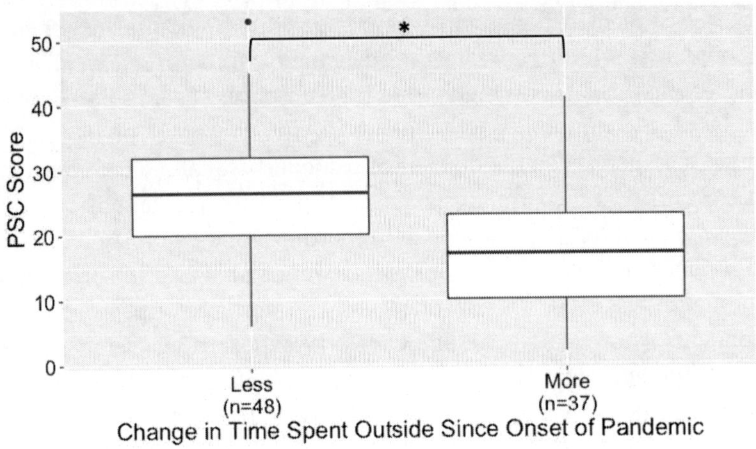

Figure 1. Distribution of PSC scores in children based on whether they reported spending less or more time outdoors since the onset of the pandemic. The asterisk indicates that the PSC scores were significantly different between the two categories ($p < 0.05$).

We then compared the PSC score distributions between parents who indicated that their child spent less time outside after the onset of the pandemic and those who reported more time spent outside (see Figure 1). For children whose parents reported that they spent less time outside ($n = 48$) following the onset of the pandemic, the range of corresponding PSC scores was 6 to 53, with a median of 27. For those who were reported to have spent more time outside ($n = 37$) following the onset of the pandemic, the PSC score range was 2 to 41, with a median of 17. Children who spent more time outside had a statistically significant ($p < 0.001$) lower distribution of PSC scores than those who spent less time outside after the onset of the pandemic.

We found that as the reported amount of time spent outside during the pandemic increased, there was a corresponding downward trend in PSC score. PSC scores were significantly lower ($p < 0.001$) for children who spent over four hours outside during the COVID months (average PSC Score of 9) compared to those who spent less than one hour outside (average PSC score of 26.5) (see Figure 2). The average PSC scores for the "Less than 1", "1-3", "3-4", and "Greater than 4" time intervals were 27, 21, 22, and 9, respectively. However, there was no statistically significant difference in the PSC score distributions between respondents who considered their neighborhood walkable ($n = 57$) versus not walkable ($n = 37$) (results not shown).

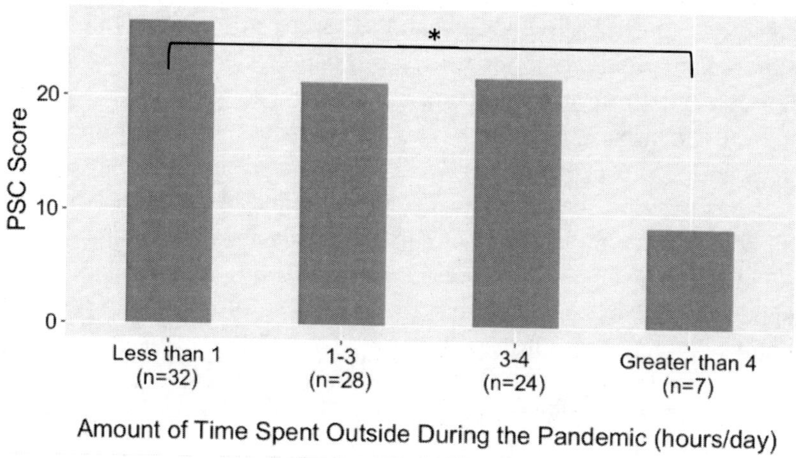

Figure 2. Average PSC scores of children based on the number of hours per day that they spent outdoors during the COVID-19 pandemic. The asterisk indicates a statistically significant difference between the average PSC scores of those who spent less than one hour outdoors and those that spent greater than four hours outdoors.

Comparing responses in higher-income and lower-income zip codes

We then compared survey responses based on whether the participant resided in a zip code that was categorized as higher-income vs lower-income. In the higher-income zip codes, 46% of the 65 respondents that reported a change in the amount of time their child spent outside during the pandemic, indicated that their child spent more time outside. Similarly, in lower-income zip codes, half of the respondents (of the 30 reporting a change) estimated more time outside during the pandemic. In the survey, walkability was described as the extent to which the urban environment is pedestrian friendly. A few examples of factors that make an environment "un-walkable" would be a lack of sidewalks, no direct path to walk to the intended location, [or] feeling that it is unsafe to walk. We did not find a statistically significant difference between perceived walkability between higher-income and lower-income zip codes. Sixty-one percent of higher-income zip code respondents indicated that their neighborhoods were walkable, and 39% reported that they felt their neighborhoods were not walkable. Approximately 58% of the respondents living in the lower-income zip code indicated that their neighborhoods were walkable, while 42% reported that they were not walkable. Looking at differences in proximity to the nearest greenspace based on walkability, 54% of respondents from higher-income zip codes reported that their children's preferred greenspaces were less than a five-minute walk from their homes, versus 40% of lower-income zip code respondents. Twenty-eight percent of lower-income zip code respondents, compared to 18% of higher-income zip code respondents, indicated having to walk between 10-20 minutes. Finally, 32% of lower-income zip code respondents and 28% higher-income zip code respondents reported needing to walk more than 20 minutes to access their children's preferred greenspaces.

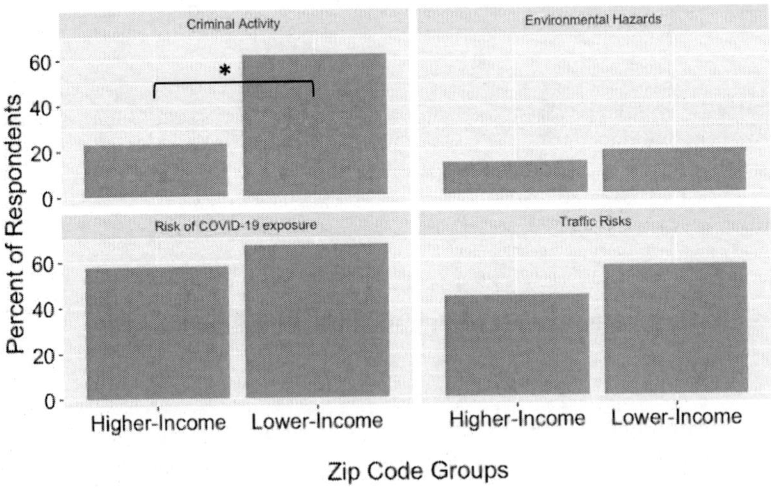

Figure 3. The percent of respondents from higher- or lower-income zip codes that selected the respective safety concern for accessing their child's preferred greenspace. There was a statistically significant difference between the percentage of higher-income and lower-income respondents that marked criminal activity, as indicated by the asterisk ($p < 0.05$).

A question about safety in greenspaces was posed through a multiple-choice list. Lower-income respondents marked a greater number of safety concerns related to accessing public greenspaces than higher-income respondents. We found a statistically significant difference in concern for criminal activity in greenspaces ($p = 0.003$), which was only viewed as a safety concern by 23% of higher-income respondents, but was reported for 62% of lower-income respondents (see Figure 3). Although risk of COVID-19 exposure or traffic risks were reported by a higher proportion of parents in lower-income zip codes, the differences in safety concerns were not statistically significant (p = 0.65 and p = 0.43, respectively). Compared to other safety concerns, environmental hazards were reported infrequently by parents as a barrier to greenspace access in both lower- and higher-income zip codes; statistical analysis evaluating differences between zip codes were not performed due to the limited proportion of parents reporting this concern. Finally, looking at mental health implications between the groups, respondents from the lower-income zip codes had a lower overall PSC distribution for their children compared to the higher-income zip codes. The range of PSC scores for children residing in the higher-income zip codes was 2 to 53, with a median of 22. The corresponding range for the lower-income zip code zip codes was 8 to 43, with a median score of 12. We found a significant difference (p = 0.02) in the distribution of PSC scores between the two groups (see Figure 4).

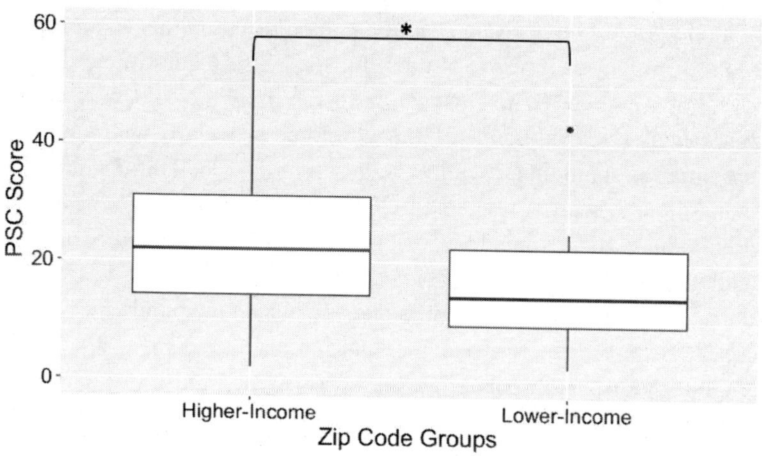

Figure 4. Distribution of PSC scores in children based on whether they lived in a high income or low income zip code. The asterisk indicates that the PSC score distribution was significantly different ($p < 0.05$) between the two categories.

Discussion

For this study, we hypothesized that the guidelines set in place due to COVID-19 would decrease the amount of time that children spent in greenspaces, and that there would be an inverse association between household income and structural barriers to greenspace, and a positive correlation between more time spent in greenspaces and better mental well-being among children. The survey data did illustrate a significant change in the amount of time that children spent outdoors due to the onset of the pandemic. However, contrary to our expectation that children would spend less time outside, approximately half of the parents indicated that their children spent more time outside after the onset of the pandemic. It should be noted that the three response options for this question were "Less time outside", "More time outside", or "Unsure". We excluded the option to choose "about the same" when answering this question because participants could indicate this outcome in the previous question that collected information on time intervals spent outdoors before and during the COVID-19 pandemic. We additionally investigated the types of greenspaces that children were using pre-pandemic and during the pandemic. When asked to indicate where their child predominately spent time outside prior to the onset of COVID-19, most parents indicated public greenspaces. During the pandemic, there was a shift away from these public spaces, which could be associated with public health restrictions, to children mainly spending outside time in the front or back yards of their homes. This, in addition to the fact that many schools converted to virtual platforms, may explain why time spent outdoors increased for many of the children, especially with the reported increase in time spent their own front or backyards. Finally, to understand how parental safety concerns related to COVID-19 exposure may have changed children's time spent outside, we looked more closely at the subgroup of respondents that specifically chose COVID-19 exposure as a reason that their child's preferred greenspace might be unsafe during the pandemic. Within this group, there were more respondents who indicated that their child spent less time outside during the pandemic than those who said more (57% vs 43% respectively). This could suggest that parents' concern for COVID-19 exposure may have played a role in the amount of time that children spent in greenspaces since going to public spaces would put them at greater risk of encountering other people, and therefore increase the risk of catching the virus. Other factors contributing to spending more time indoors and less time outdoors reported through the survey included reduced outdoor activities such as organized sports, greenspace closures, and halted public transportation to greenspaces. Walkability was an aspect considered throughout the study as well, however, when looking at factors that contributed to changed time spent outdoors due to the onset of the pandemic, it may not have been important since we also saw an increase in time spent in front or back yards, for which walkability would not be a relevant factor.

To examine the relationships between these changes and perceived mental health in children, we first compared whether parents indicated that their children spent more or less time outside during the pandemic with their respective PSC scores. We found a statistically significant difference between the two categories indicating that children who increased the time spent outdoors during the pandemic had lower PSC scores than those who reduced their time spent outdoors during the pandemic. This lower PSC score distribution supports previous data (4, 18), suggesting better mental health in children who spend more time outside. To further explore the relationship between time spent outside and mental health, we compared the estimated time spent outside during the pandemic and the average PSC scores associated with each time interval. We found a clear downward trend in PSC score, thus indicating better mental health, as kids spent more time outdoors. Moreover, there was a 67% decrease in average scores of children spending less than one hour outside and those spending more than four hours outside. This supports a correlation between children spending time outside and better mental well-being as reported by their parents. Asking parents to report their child's age in addition to filling out the PSC would have provided stronger data regarding its application to questions correlating time spent in greenspace and mental well-being since the checklist is particularly designed for children between the ages of 4 and 17 years (12).

To assess some of the socioeconomic barriers to accessing greenspace, we used the respondents' reported zip code data to categorize them into higher- or lower-income zip codes. We did not find a significant difference in the changes to their outdoor activities, nor in the perceived walkability between the higher-income and lower-income zip codes. Similar studies in Seattle, San Diego, and Tucson found higher-income neighborhoods to be in closer proximity to preferred greenspaces or have easier access to them by a direct, walkable path (5, 6). While our results addressing this topic were not statistically different, 54% of higher-income zip code respondents reported that the nearest walkable greenspace was less than a 5-minute walk, whereas only 40% of the lower-income zip code respondents indicated that the nearest walkable greenspace was less than a 5-minute walk. Similarly, a greater percentage of lower-income zip code respondents (60%) indicated having to walk more than 10 minutes to access greenspace compared to the higher-income zip code respondents (46%). These differences were not statistically significant, but this may be a factor of our small sample population. If true, this may suggest that residents of higher-income neighborhoods in Durham may be in closer proximity to preferred greenspaces or have easier access to them, specifically regarding a direct, walkable path. In light of COVID-19 and the increased reports that children were spending more time at home, less frequently accessing public greenspaces, and spending more time in their front and backyards, walkability was not as relevant in assessing access to greenspace. Still, it is worth conducting further research on walkability within Durham County as it can provide data on neighborhood characteristics that may be important in understanding structural barriers to local greenspaces.

Exploring the idea of equitable access further, we considered factors such as perceived neighborhood safety concerns, which could act as barriers for children to visit public greenspaces. When completing the survey, parents were able to select any combination of the following concerns: risk of COVID-19 exposure, traffic risks, environmental hazards, and criminal activity. There was a significantly greater concern for neighborhood criminal activity in lower-income zip codes compared to HI, and while differences were not statistically significant, a greater proportion of parents in lower-income zip codes also reported COVID-19 and traffic concerns. Previous research found that improved safety factors and lower crime, as well as aesthetics, were associated with more frequent activity in nearby parks, thus supporting our finding that concern for neighborhood criminal activity is likely a social factor that impacts the use of greenspaces in Durham (5, 19).

Finally, we found that the lower-income zip code respondents had a PSC score distribution that was significantly lower than that of the higher-income zip codes. This contradicted our hypothesis, indicating that children living in lower-income neighborhoods had better mental health than those from higher-income neighborhoods. Despite the correlations between time spent outdoors and better mental health, as well as proximity to greenspaces, respondents from lower-income neighborhoods reported fewer psychosocial behaviors that would indicate poor mental well-being. Social and economic factors including but not limited to age, race, and whether or not school was conducted in-person or virtually, may have acted as confounding variables; however, we were unable to adjust for these variables. Another element to consider is that those living in higher-income zip codes may have better access to mental health services, and therefore may be more aware and attuned to their children's mental health, activities, and behaviors (20, 21). Further, parents, in addition to their children, experienced novel stressors as a result of the COVID-19 pandemic. This included, but was not limited to drastic changes in work for many parents. For some this involved going to jobs with the daily risk of exposure to the virus, for others this may have included transitioning to working from home or even being without work. In this study, the PSC scores recorded reflect parents' perceptions of their children's behaviors and mental well-being, thus there is inherent possibility for the mental status of parents to influence PSC scores. Due to the limitations of the study, however, further analysis would need to be conducted to more accurately analyze the mental health status of children within these groups.

Strengths and limitations

There were many limitations to this study. First, we had a limited sample size, including a predominantly white sample from mostly higher-income zip codes, which is not representative of the Durham population. There was also possible non-response bias, in which participation was limited by the necessity to access technology and spend time filling out a lengthy online survey (22). This skew in the participating population towards those who were English speaking, had internet access, digital literacy, and access to social media sites may have contributed to the disproportionate percentage of respondents coming from higher-income zip codes. Nonetheless, the number of respondents provided enough power to conduct some limited statistical analysis.

Since the survey was conducted retrospectively, in pre-COVID-19 and during-COVID-19 time periods, there was also the possibility that recall bias may have influenced the validity of the results. However, using social media, we were able to reach parents during a pandemic and receive prompt feedback on their children's behaviors, activities, and mental health awareness. Regarding limitations within the survey, we did not ask parents to report the age of the child they were referencing when filling out the survey. Having this data would have given us a better understanding about how greenspace is being used (actively or passively) in the context of their responses. Age also would have helped us determine how to accurately apply the PSC, which was designed for the particular age group of 4 to 17 years old. Additionally, there may have been cases in which parents were filling out the survey for children younger than school age, where time spent outside would not have been accurately defined by the options given in the survey. Social conformity bias may have also influenced survey responses to survey questions regarding children's reported time spent outside (i.e., perceptions that more time outdoors is preferred, thus leading to over-reporting). Further, the use of zip codes as an indicator for income status is a limitation since we used a community variable as a proxy for individual level information. Finally, we were unable to adjust for individual variables that may have confounded analyses, such as age and race as discussed previously.

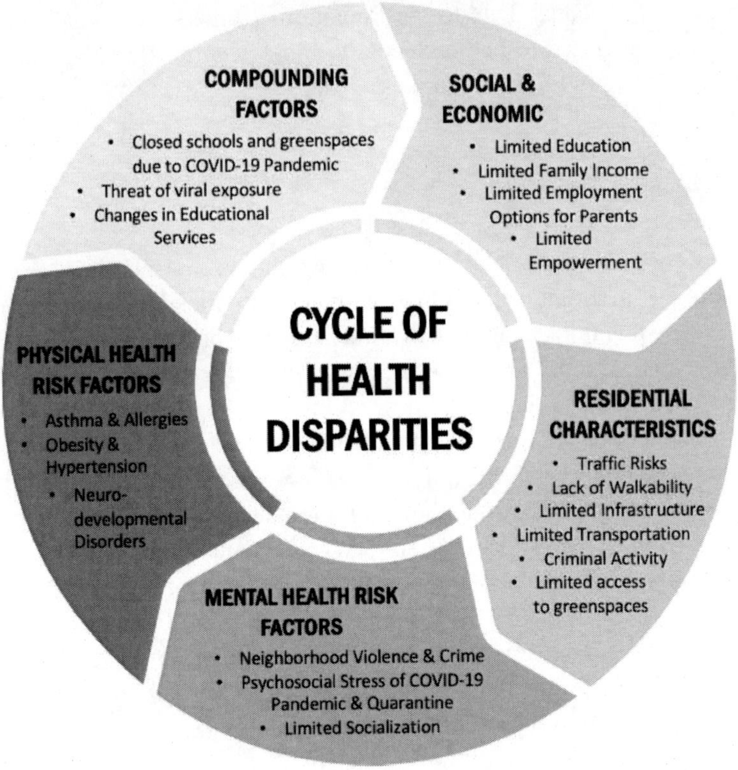

Figure 5. The cycle of health disparities that results from differential exposure to adverse environmental factors and can impact children's physical and mental health.

Conclusion

Health disparities are outcomes which result from differential exposure to adverse environmental factors by some populations compared to others, and can have significant impacts on the health and wellbeing of children (23). The intersection of these disparities can be visualized as a cycle (see Figure 5). Social and economic stressors are often paired with poorer conditions in the surrounding built environment and natural environment. These stressors may lead to limitations in income opportunities for families, quality education, transportation, and more (7, 23). Consequently, children suffer physically and mentally. Barriers to health prevent children from thriving within their environments, and the cycle continues. In regard to the topics explored in this research, there are many ways in which barriers to accessing greenspace during the COVID-19 pandemic could contribute to this cycle (see Figure 5). For example, lack of sidewalks and traffic risks limit children's ability to walk to public greenspaces when transportation is not available (3). Characteristics such as neighborhood criminal activity may create barriers to greenspace access and impact overall health (3, 6).

The onset of the COVID-19 pandemic and the consequent stay-at-home orders not only exacerbated these preexisting issues by increasing the amount of time that children spent in neighborhoods where they face potential environmental health risks, but also introduced new stressors (9). A few examples of these added stressors include reduced access to educational resources during the pandemic, e.g., direct contact with educators, access to tools such as books or technology provided at schools, etc., limited social interactions with peers due to restrictions on social gathering for school or leisure, and a lack of diversity in their social environments. In households where parents faced lost income due to the dramatic unemployment rate early in the pandemic, additional stressors such as financial insecurity and food insecurity may have increased children's psychosocial stress and adversely impacted mental well-being (24, 25). This project aimed to identify what role that greenspace plays in improving mental health for children and to identify which socioeconomic factors act as obstacles to accessing those greenspaces, with the intention of creating proposed action steps for minimizing these hurdles.

Indeed, we identified a strong association between time spent outdoors and children's mental well-being, and we identified barriers in access to greenspace that varied by community income. While the results of this study did not suggest that economic disparities influenced children's mental well-being, there is still much to investigate regarding the pandemic's impact on children's well-being and related health disparities. This research can provide a useful starting point for communities in Durham to work together to increase the amount of time children spend outdoors given the ongoing pandemic. Additionally, it may contribute to identifying ways to "break the cycle" of health disparities by highlighting concerns related to criminal activity in greenspaces. Future research should further investigate how a child's age factors into the association between time spent outdoors and mental well-being, in order to more definitely establish this association and develop effective interventions by age group. By creating safer and more accessible greenspaces in Durham neighborhoods, we hope to contribute to the goal of improving children's mental well-being within the community.

Acknowledgments

I would like to thank all the families in Durham, NC who participated in this study. Also, thank you to Roshen Amin for his help with statistical analysis and designing figures. Finally, we thank the BTC Program faculty for their support and for giving me a platform to explore my interests in environmental children's health within my local community.

References

[1] Oxford. Greenspace definition. Lexico 2021. URL: https://www.lexico.com/en/definition/green_space.

[2] Mitra R, Moore SA, Gillespie M, Faulkner G, Vanderloo LM, Chulak-Bozzer T, et al. Healthy movement behaviours in children and youth during the COVID-19 pandemic: Exploring the role of the neighbourhood environment. Health Place 2020;65:102418. doi: https://doi.org/10.1016/j.healthplace.2020.102418.

[3] Uchiyama Y, Kohsaka R. Access and use of green areas during the COVID-19 pandemic: Green infrastructure management in the "new normal". Sustainability 2020;12(23):9842. doi: https://doi.org/10.3390/su12239842.

[4] McCormick R. Does access to green space impact the mental well-being of children: A systematic review. J Pediatr Nurs 2017;37:3–7. doi: https://doi.org/10.1016/j.pedn.2017.08.027.

[5] Tappe KA, Glanz K, Sallis JF, Zhou C, Saelens BE. Children's physical activity and parents' perception of the neighborhood environment: Neighborhood impact on kids study. Int J Behav Nutr Phys Act 2013;10:39. doi: https://doi.org/10.1186/1479-5868-10-39.

[6] Zuniga-Teran AA, Stoker P, Gimblett RH, Orr BJ, Marsh SE, Guertin DP, et al. Exploring the influence of neighborhood walkability on the frequency of use of greenspace. Landsc Urban Plan 2019;190:103609. doi: https://doi.org/10.1016/j.landurbplan.2019.103609.

[7] Shumow L, Vandell DL, Posner J. Risk and resilience in the urban neighborhood: Predictors of academic performance among low-income elementary school children. Merrill Palmer Q 1999;45(2):309–31.

[8] AJMC Staff. A timeline of COVID-19 developments in 2020. AJMC 2021. URL: https://www.ajmc.com/view/a-timeline-of-covid19-developments-in-2020.

[9] Lancker WV, Parolin Z. COVID-19, school closures, and child poverty: A social crisis in the making. Lancet Public Health 2020;5(5):e243-4. doi: https://doi.org/10.1016/S2468-2667(20)30084-0.

[10] Golberstein E, Wen H, Miller BF. Coronavirus disease 2019 (COVID-19) and mental health for children and adolescents. JAMA Pediatr 2020;174(9):819. doi: https://doi.org/10.1001/jamapediatrics.2020.1456.

[11] Tulchin-Francis K, Stevens W, Gu X, Zhang T, Roberts H, Keller J, et al. The impact of the coronavirus disease 2019 pandemic on physical activity in US children. J Sport Health Sci 2021;10(3):323–32. doi: https://doi.org/10.1016/j.jshs.2021.02.005.

[12] Pediatric symptom checklist. Massachusetts General Hospital. URL: https://www.massgeneral.org/psychiatry/treatments-and-services/pediatric-symptom-checklist

[13] Jellinek M, Little M, Murphy JM, Pagano M. The Pediatric symptom checklist: Support for a role in a managed care environment. Arch Pediatr Adolesc Med 1995;149(7):740–6. doi: https://doi.org/10.1001/archpedi.1995.02170200030004.

[14] Jellinek MS, Murphy JM, Little M, Pagano ME, Comer DM, Kelleher KJ. Use of the pediatric symptom checklist to screen for psychosocial problems in pediatric primary care: A national feasibility study. Arch Pediatr Adolesc Med 1999;153(3):254–60. doi: https://doi.org/10.1001/archpedi.153.3.254.

[15] Durham NC profile: Facts and data, 2020. URL: https://northcarolina.hometownlocator.com/nc/durham/durham.cfm.

[16] Zipcodes in Durham county. Zipdatamaps.Com 2021. URL: https://zipdatamaps.com.

[17] Durham NC demographics. World Population Review 2021. URL: https://worldpopulationreview.com/us-cities/durham-nc-population.

[18] Fyfe-Johnson AL, Marcuse EK, Tandon P, Hazlehurst M, Bratman GN, Thomas R, et al. Nature and children's health: A systematic review. Pediatrics 2021; 148(4):e2020049155. doi: 10.1542/peds.2020-049155.

[19] Gold S. Nonuse of neighborhood parks. J Am Inst Plann 1972;38(6):369-78. doi: 10.1080/01944367208977640.

[20] Vukojević M, Zovko Grbeša A, Talić I, Tanović M, Rešić B, Vrdoljak I, et al. Parental socioeconomic status as a predictor of physical and mental health outcomes in children—literature review. Acta Clin Croat 2017;56:742–8. doi: https://doi.org/10.20471/acc.2017.56.04.23.

[21] Cummings JR, Allen L, Clennon J, Ji X, Druss BG. Geographic access to specialty mental health care across high- and low-income US communities. JAMA Psychiatry 2017;74(5):476–84. doi: https://doi.org/10.1001/jamapsychiatry.2017.0303.

[22] Prince M. 9—Epidemiology. In: Wright P, Stern J, Phelan M, eds. Core Psychiatry 2012;3:115–29. doi: https://doi.org/10.1016/B978-0-7020-3397-1.00009-4.

[23] Rubin L, Geller R, Coles CD, Greeen V, Mutic A, Mutic N, et al. Break the cycle of children's environmental health disparities: 14th Annual review of program and student projects. Int J Child Health Hum Dev 2019;12(4):283-99.

[24] Knowles M, Rabinowich J, Ettinger de Cuba S, Cutts DB, Chilton M. "Do you wanna breathe or eat?": Parent perspectives on child health consequences of food insecurity, trade-offs, and toxic stress. Matern Child Health J 2016;20(1):25–32. doi: https://doi.org/10.1007/s10995-015-1797-8.

[25] Kuruvilla A, Jacob K. Poverty, social stress and mental health. Indian J Med Res 2007;126:273–8.

Chapter 8

Neighborhood quality and positive health indicators among urban adolescents

Han N Oo[1,*], Miranda Spratlen[1], MHS, PhD, Courtney K Blackwell[2], PhD, Teresa Durham[1], Jia Guo[3], MS, PhD, Lori Hoepner[1], MPH, DrPh, Diurka Diaz[1], MA, Gladys Badia[1], MA, Shuang Wang[4], PhD and Julie B Herbstman[1], MSc, PhD

[1]Department of Environmental Health Sciences, Columbia University Mailman School of Public Health, New York, United States of America

[2]Department of Medical Social Sciences, Northwestern University, Chicago, Illinois, United States of America

[3]Department of Psychiatry, Columbia University, New York, United States of America

[4]Department of Biostatistics, Columbia University, New York, United States of America

Abstract

There is a growing epidemiologic interest to expand the scope of health research beyond disease and risk factors to a more comprehensive evaluation of all health states, including those on the positive end of the spectrum ("positive health"). Neighborhood quality (NQ) is a potentially modifiable factor that may influence positive health. We evaluated the association between perception of NQ in childhood and indicators of positive health among adolescents who live in low-income, urban neighborhoods of New York City. Mothers assessed NQ prospectively via questionnaire at child ages 5, 7, 9, and 11 years. Indicators of positive health domains including general health, physical health, and mental health were assessed and reported by mothers when their children were

* *Correspondence:* Han N Oo, PrIMER Trainee, Department of Environmental Health Sciences, Columbia University, 722 W 168th St, New York, NY 10032, United States. Email: hoo1@fordham.edu.

between the ages of 10-20 years and self-reported among a subset of children at 16-20 years. Children were grouped into "stressed" and "non-stressed" NQ groups based on the repeated prospective maternal report evaluating various aspects of their neighborhood. Overall, we found a general trend that those in the perceived "non-stressed" NQ groups had better Global Health compared to those in the "stressed" NQ group. In the subset of children who provided self-report, we observed significant associations between better overall NQ and NQ safety and better Global Health. We also observed a significant relationship between greater perceived neighborhood social cohesion and lower psychological stress. Our findings identify an important modifiable environmental factor in child and adolescent health that could serve as a focus for interventions to help break the cycle of children's environmental health disparities.

Introduction

There is a growing interest in the epidemiologic landscape to expand the scope of health research beyond disease and risk factors to a more comprehensive evaluation of all health states, including those on the positive end of the spectrum (1). Identification of risk factors for disease and negative health outcomes remains essential; however, focusing only on these health attributes fails to fully capture the broad range of social, emotional, and physical health. In turn, this leaves a gap in our understanding of the factors that are associated with better health outcomes beyond "non-diseased" and indicative of better quality of life.

Healthy People 2020 underscored this shift in focus solely on traditional indicators of population health, such as life expectancy and causes of death, to a more expansive assessment of health aimed at characterizing health related quality of life (HRQoL) and well-being (2). Well-being indicators are designed to measure positive experiences in people's daily lives such as positive emotions, resilience, realization of potential and life satisfaction (3). Mounting evidence demonstrates the importance of these positive health indicators as both predictors and outcomes in health research, with effect sizes comparable to more traditional risk factors (1). For example, a meta-analysis of longitudinal studies found that both purpose in life and life satisfaction were independently associated with up to 25% reductions in mortality risk (4, 5). In addition, positive emotions have been associated with numerous domains of physical health, including better immune functioning, decreased risk of disease and injury, and better self-reported health (6). Further, the absence of health problems does not equate to the presence of well-being (7), suggesting incremental utility of evaluating an individual's positive health. Positive health research has been defined as "promoting an understanding of the developmental pathways for those biological, functional, behavioral, and experiential health assets that promote goal attainment and needs satisfaction as well as individuals' subjective experiences of life as happy, satisfying, and meaningful (i.e., well-being)" (8).

Understanding predictors of positive health is as important as understanding predictors of disease or dysfunction. Neighborhood quality (NQ) is a potentially modifiable factor that may influence the positive health construct. There is a substantial evidence base relating significant effects of neighborhoods on both adult (9-13) and child health (14–17), including defining neighborhoods physically (e.g., access to green space), objectively (e.g., socioeconomic status), as well as subjectively (e.g., participant neighborhood perception). Studies also suggest that perceived neighborhood quality is more strongly associated with health than objective neighborhood indicators and may mediate the association between these objective neighborhood measures and health outcomes (12, 13). Several studies have reported a significant relationship between perceived neighborhood quality and positive health/quality of life among adults (18–22), but less is known about this relationship among adolescents (23).

In this study, we evaluated the association between perceived neighborhood quality and four indicators of positive health (life satisfaction, global health, sleep disturbance and psychological stress), in adolescents who live in low-income, urban neighborhoods of New York City.

Our study

The subjects for the study were participants from the Mothers and Newborns Study which is a prospective longitudinal birth cohort comprised of mother-child dyads at the Columbia Center for Children's Environmental Health (CCCEH) (24). Women (n=727) from ages 18 to 35-year-olds were recruited into the study from the prenatal clinics around CCCEH which included the New York Presbyterian Medical Center, Harlem Hospital, and their satellite clinics. Participants were Dominican and African American women. They resided in Northern Manhattan (Washington Heights, Central Harlem) or the South Bronx. Women who smoked, used illicit drugs, had pre-existing conditions such as diabetes, hypertension, or known HIV infection were excluded from the study. Women who had their first prenatal visit after the 20th week of pregnancy were also excluded from the study. The study received approval from the Institutional Review Board of Columbia University. The participants provided informed consent after learning about all study procedures.

Exposure measure

The 32-item Neighborhood Quality Assessment (25–27) is comprised of a questionnaire that was conducted when children were 5, 7, 9 and 11 years old and intended to evaluate patterns of neighborhood quality (NQ) over time across middle childhood. The questionnaire generated a total NQ score and also included subscales to measure different aspects of NQ. The first sub-scale is social order/disorder. An example statement is "the neighborhood streets are busy with shoppers, mothers with strollers, and children playing." The second subscale is safety and violence. For this subscale, the mothers are asked how worried they are about certain situations in the neighborhood. An example is "how worried they are about letting their children go outside during the night." The last sub-scale is social cohesion and neighborhood stability. An example statement is "the people moving into the neighborhood in the past year or so are good for the neighborhood." Items in the first two subscales were measured using the 0-4 Likert Scale. Items in the last subscale were measured as a yes or a no.

The assessment was conducted in three steps, as described previously (28). Briefly, in Step 1, a 32-question self-reported NQ questionnaire was administered to the participants. In Step 2, each participant's total NQ score and three individual subscale scores were standardized and scaled for the presence of neighborhood "stress." In Step 3, trajectory models were fit using the method described in Durham et al. (28) We used finite mixture models to develop trajectories of total and individual subscale scores and selected the best fitting model for each NQ outcome (total NQ, social order/disorder, safety and violence, and social cohesion and neighborhood stability) using the Bayesian Information Criterion (BIC). These analyses were conducted using the SAS Proc Traj macro (28). Proc TRAJ uses any data provided to include the individual in the model that best fits them. Individuals need not have all data points to be included. The trajectory models helped to create these two neighborhood quality groups: stressed and non-stressed.

Outcome measure

Three measures were used to assess positive health. The Patient-Reported Outcomes Measurement Information System (PROMIS®) Parent-Proxy Global Health measure was used for the parent's report of their child's positive health (29). The proxy asks seven questions regarding a child's general health, quality of life, physical health, mental health, emotions, and social skills. Mothers reported on behalf of their children (n=528). The answer choices range from excellent [5] to poor [1]. The second measure was the Child PROMIS Pediatric Global Health measure which provides a self-assessment of the child's physical, mental, and social health and has parallel items to the parent-proxy version. This scale was administered to a random subset of children (n=62) who were over 16-20 years of age. For both maternal and child report of Global Health scales, sums were calculated for subscales and higher scores indicate better positive health. The third measure was the ECHO Positive Health Outcomes parent report, which is composed of PROMIS instruments: PROMIS Parent-Proxy Life Satisfaction (four questions) (n=408), Sleep Disturbance (4 questions) (n=408), and Psychological Stress Experience (4 questions) (n=407). Sums were calculated for each subscale and lower scores indicate better positive health for the stress and sleep domains whereas higher scores indicate better positive health for the life satisfaction and meaning and purpose domains. All assessments were administered either by phone or via secure texted link. All PROMIS measures were transformed to T-scores (with mean=50 and SD=10) using the standard PROMIS scoring procedures (30). All PROMIS measures used in the current study were calibrated and normed using large reference populations, representative of the general US population.

Sociodemographic measures

Maternal education and ethnicity were obtained during the prenatal baseline questionnaire. Child sex was abstracted from the medical record at birth.

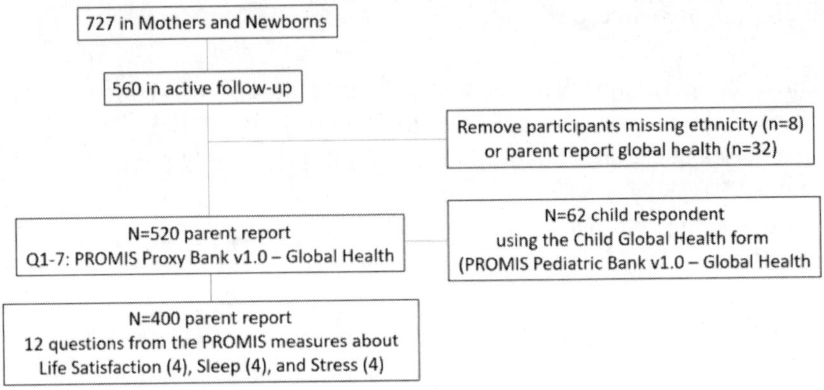

Figure 1. Flow chart of the participants.

Statistical approach

For study analyses, we included participants who had complete data on maternal education and ethnicity; child age, gender; NQ indicators; and outcome measures (Parent Proxy Global Health, Sleep Disturbance, Psychological Stress Experience and Life Satisfactions Scales), resulting in a sample size of 400 (see Figure 1). Medians (IQR) were used to evaluate differences in T-scores for our outcome measures by sociodemographic and NQ indicator variables. Significance of differences were calculated using Kruskal-Wallis tests.

We used exploratory data analyses to assess distributions of both independent and dependent variables. Both parent proxy and child self-report Global Health T-scores were normally distributed and were therefore analyzed as continuous variables. To compare Global Health scores between the subset of participants with both maternal report and child self-report (n=60), we used a paired t-test and calculated a Pearson correlation. Linear regression was used with an interaction term between maternal report and age to determine if the relationship between child self-report and maternal report varied with age. Due to the non-normality of T-scores for sleep disturbance, psychological stress experience and life satisfaction outcomes, we dichotomized these scales based on established PROMIS score cut-points (see Table 1). For life satisfaction, the reference group (n=49) included participants in the low/very low life satisfaction category and the non-reference group (n=351) included participants in the average or higher categories (in this study, no participants reported life satisfaction higher than average). For sleep disturbance, the reference group (n=270) included participants in the normal sleep disturbance category and the non-reference group (n=130) included participants in the mild, moderate and severe sleep disturbance categories. For psychological stress experience, the reference group (n=157) included participants in the low or very low stress categories and the non-reference group (n=243) included participants in the average or higher stress categories.

Table 1. PROMIS scale cut points

Category	Count (%)
Life Satisfaction	
Categorical	
Very Low	4 (1.0)
Low	45(11.2)
Average	351 (87.8)
High	0
Very High	0
Dichotomized	
Low/Very Low	49 (12.2)
Average+	351 (87.8)
Sleep Disturbance	
Categorical	
Normal	270 (67.5)
Mild	38 (9.5)
Moderate	24 (6.0)
Severe	68 (17)
Dichotomized	
Normal	270 (67.5)
Disturbed	130 (32.5)
Psychological Stress Experience	
Categorical	
Very Low	0
Low	157 (39.2)
Average	174 (43.5)
High	52 (13.0)
Very High	17 (4.2)
Dichotomized	
Low	157 (39.2)
Average+	243 (60.8)

We used separate linear regression models to evaluate the association between dichotomous NQ indicators (not stressed vs. stressed) and Parent Proxy Global Health T-scores. We used separate logistic regression models to evaluate the association between NQ indicators and dichotomous outcomes (sleep disturbance, psychological stress experience and life satisfaction). All adjusted models were controlled for child age and sex and maternal ethnicity and education.

Software

All figures and analyses were conducted using R Version 1.4.1106.

Our findings

Among the 400 children of mothers included in this study, the median age for PROMIS scales was 16.4 years and the median for the PROMIS Parent Proxy Global Health Scale was 16.1 years (see Table 2). There were slightly more

Table 2. Bivariate associations of PROMIS scales by sociodemographics and neighborhood quality scales

	Parent Proxy Global		Life Satisfaction		Stress		Sleep Disturbance	
	Median (IQR)	p-value	Median (IQR)	p-value	Median (IQR)	p-value	Median (IQR)	p-value
Age (PROMIS)								
<=16.36	44.6 (37.4, 51.4)	0.703	49.8 (42.6, 59.2)	0.764	46.5 (39.6, 55.7)	0.048	47.1 (47.1, 58.0)	0.8
>16.36	44.7 (37.2, 51.2)		48.1 (42.6, 59.2)		49.2 (39.6, 58.2)		47.1 (47.1, 58.0)	
Age (Global)								
<=16.09	45.2 (37.9, 51.5)	0.361	49.8 (42.6, 59.2)	0.579	46.5 (39.6, 55.9)	0.094	47.1 (47.1, 58.0)	0.634
>16.09	44.2 (36.8, 51.2)		48.1 (42.6, 59.2)		49.0 (39.6, 58.2)		47.1 (47.1, 58.2)	
Gender								
Female	44.1 (37.4, 51.5)	0.788	48.5 (42.6, 59.2)	0.639	49.1 (39.6, 58.2)	0.042	47.1 (47.1, 57.9)	0.623
Male	45.2 (37.2, 51.0)		49.9 (42.6, 59.2)		46.5 (39.6, 55.6)		47.1 (47.1, 60.6)	
Ethnicity								
African American	45.1 (38, 51.4)	0.23	52.4 (42.6, 59.2)	0.013	49.0 (39.6, 58.2)	0.654	47.1 (47.1, 55.9)	0.089
Dominican/Dominican American	44.2 (36.8, 50.9)		48.1 (42.6, 59.2)		47.0 (39.6, 56.1)		47.1 (47.1, 59.8)	
Education								
<High School	43.8 (37.3, 51.9)	0.946	49.8 (42.6, 59.2)	0.697	47.5 (39.6, 55.7)	0.27	47.1 (47.1, 57.9)	0.855
High School/GED	44.9 (37.4, 51.2)		48.1 (42.6, 59.2)		47.6 (39.6, 58.1)		47.1 (47.1, 58)	
>High School	45.2 (36.8, 51.0)		48.1 (42.6, 59.2)		49.2 (39.6, 56.7)		47.1 (47.1, 58.6)	
Group All								
Non-stressed	45.0 (37.2, 51.3)	0.578	50.5 (42.6, 59.2)	0.286	47.0 (39.6, 56.1)	0.286	47.1 (47.1, 57.9)	0.261
Stressed	43.8 (37.4, 51.3)		48.1 (42.6, 59.2)		49.0 (39.6, 56.1)		47.1 (47.1, 60.1)	
Group Order								
Non-stressed	45.0 (37, 51.25)	0.684	48.5 (42.6, 59.2)	0.948	47.5 (39.6, 56.1)	0.363	47.1 (47.1, 57.9)	0.136
Stressed	43.8 (37.5, 51.4)		48.8 (42.6, 59.2)		49.0 (39.6, 56.1)		47.1 (47.1, 62.8)	
Group Safety								
Non-stressed	45.1 (37.2, 51.3)	0.438	50.6 (42.6, 59.2)	0.163	47.6 (39.6, 57.3)	0.795	47.1 (47.1, 58.0)	0.678
Stressed	43.7 (37.2, 51.3)		48.1 (42.6, 59.2)		49 (39.6, 56.1)		47.1 (47.1, 58.4)	
Group Social								
Non-stressed	44.6 (36.8, 50.7)	0.296	49.9 (42.6, 59.2)	0.528	46.5 (39.6, 56.1)	0.15	47.1 (47.1, 58)	0.349
Stressed	45 (38.1, 52.6)		48.1 (42.6, 59.2)		49.4 (39.6, 56.1)		47.1 (47.1, 58.5)	
Total (Median (IQR))	44.7 (37.2, 51.3)		48.7 (42.6, 59.2)		47.7 (39.6, 56.1)		47.1 (47.1, 58)	
Total (Mean (SD))	44.9 (9.97)		49.4 (8.77)		49.7 (10.5)		53.0 (8.60)	

females (55%) and the majority of participants were of Dominican/Dominican American ethnicity (63.8%), with the remaining being of African American ethnicity (36.3%). Approximately one-third of mothers (37.8%) had less than a high school education, 39.5% having a high school education or equivalent, and 22.8% having greater than a high school education. The majority of participants reported living in neighborhoods that were classified as "non-stressed" neighborhood quality groups (64.3% for overall NQ, 67.8% for social order, 61.0% for safety, and 68.3% for social cohesion).

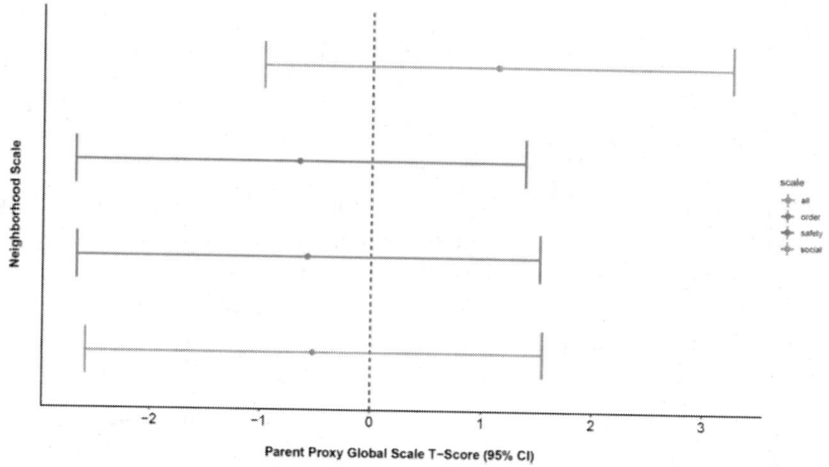

Figure 2A. Parent proxy (N=400).

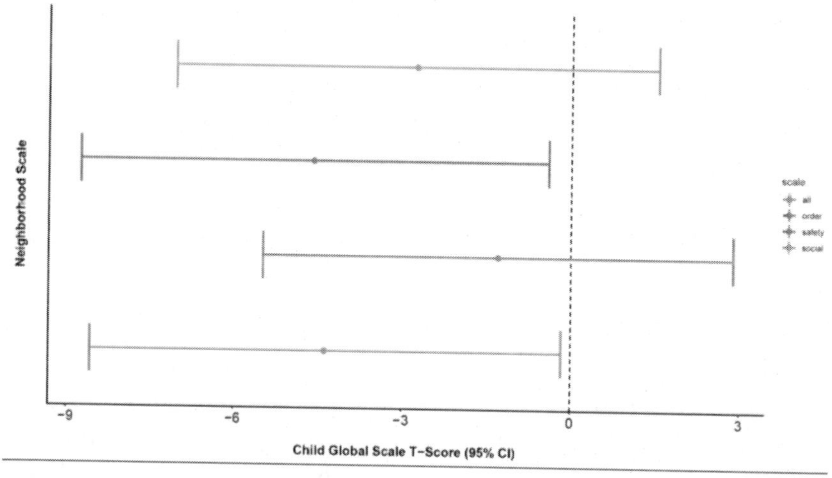

Figure 2B. Child self-report (N=52).

Figure 2. Global scores comparing stressed and non-stressed groups, controlling for child sex and age, maternal education and ethnicity.

In terms of the positive health scales, the means for both life satisfaction and psychological stress experience were very close to the general population normative average of 50 (49.4 and 49.7, respectively). The mean for the PROMIS Parent Proxy Global Health scale was slightly lower (44.9) and the mean for the sleep disturbance scale was slightly higher (53.1) than the general population average, however, both were within one standard deviation (10). Greater stress was reported among females (p=0.04) and older children (p=0.05). In addition, African Americans reported higher life satisfaction scores compared to Dominican/Dominican Americans (p=0.01).

A subset of 62 children provided a self-report of their Global Health generally 6 months after the maternal report. On average, the child's self-report was non-significantly lower than their maternal report (45.2 vs. 46.4, p=0.29). The correlation between these measures was relatively low and not statistically significant (Pearson=0.10, p = 0.44). This relationship did not vary by child age at the time of the report.

Figure 2 displays the estimates representing the difference in average Global Health T-scores comparing the stressed groups to the non-stressed groups using both the parent proxy (see Figure 2A) and the child self-report in the smaller subset (see Figure 2B), after controlling for the child's gender and age, and maternal education and ethnicity. For the parent proxy, a linear regression analysis revealed that for the overall neighborhood quality, order, and safety neighborhood scales, the estimates were negative, suggesting that children living in stressed neighborhoods scored lower on the Global Health scale compared to children living in "non-stressed" neighborhoods. However, these associations were not statistically significant. For the child self- report in the subset of n=52 (with complete demographic and child report Global Health scale data) the direction of the association was similar for overall, order, and safety subscales and statistically significant (p<0.05) for the safety and overall subscales.

Table 3 displays odds ratios and 95% confidence intervals for associations between neighborhood quality indicators (non-stressed vs. stressed) and dichotomized PROMIS sub scales (Life Satisfaction, Psychological Stress Experience and Sleep Disturbance) in both crude and adjusted models, controlling for child's age and gender and maternal ethnicity and education. In general, life satisfaction was non-significantly lower in the stressed group across all NQ indicators except for social cohesion which was close to the null. Psychological stress and sleep disturbance were typically higher in the stressed group across all NQ indicators and reached significance for social cohesion and stress (OR=1.67, 95% CI=1.06, 2.64).

Table 3. Associations (odds ratios (95% CIs)) between neighborhood quality indices and quality of life outcomes

Exposure	Life Satisfaction (+)		Stress (-)		Sleep Disturbance (-)	
	Crude	Adjusted	Crude	Adjusted	Crude	Adjusted
Group All						
Non-stressed	Reference (1.00)	Reference (1.00)	Reference (1.00)	Reference (1.00)	Reference (1.00)	Reference (1.00)
Stressed	0.59 (0.32 , 1.08)	0.61 (0.33 , 1.13)	1.33 (0.87 , 2.04)	1.40 (0.91 , 2.17)	1.38 (0.89 , 2.12)	1.37 (0.88 , 2.12)
Group Order						
Non-stressed	Reference (1.00)	Reference (1.00)	Reference (1.00)	Reference (1.00)	Reference (1.00)	Reference (1.00)
Stressed	0.59 (0.32 , 1.1)	0.62 (0.33 , 1.16)	1.38 (0.9 , 2.15)	1.43 (0.91 , 2.26)	1.44 (0.92 , 2.23)	1.53 (0.97 , 2.4)
Group Social						
Non-stressed	Reference (1.00)	Reference (1.00)	Reference (1.00)	Reference (1.00)	Reference (1.00)	Reference (1.00)
Stressed	1.06 (0.57 , 2.08)	1.05 (0.56 , 2.07)	1.63 (1.05 , 2.56)	1.67 (1.06 , 2.64)	1.28 (0.82 , 1.99)	1.28 (0.82 , 2.0)
Group Safety						
Non-stressed	Reference (1.00)	Reference (1.00)	Reference (1.00)	Reference (1.00)	Reference (1.00)	Reference (1.00)
Stressed	0.69 (0.38 , 1.27)	0.72 (0.39 , 1.33)	0.97 (0.64 , 1.46)	1.00 (0.65 , 1.52)	1.23 (0.8 , 1.88)	1.17 (0.76 , 1.81)

Adjusted for: child's gender and age, and maternal education and ethnicity.

Discussion

We conducted an analysis within a longitudinal birth cohort study including women and children living in Northern Manhattan and South Bronx to determine whether maternal report of perceived neighborhood quality during middle childhood (ages 5, 7, 9, and 11 years) was associated with "positive" health outcomes in children, including a Global Health measure, child's life satisfaction, sleep disturbance, and psychological stress experience. Our study participants did not have positive health scores that varied significantly from the PROMIS national normative sample. However, we found that children living in more stressed neighborhoods had generally lower (worse) scores on the Global Health measure than children living in non-stressed neighborhoods. When considering life satisfaction, psychological stress, and sleep disturbance scales, the relationships were similar and only statistically significant when comparing children living in neighborhoods with more social cohesion to those living in neighborhoods with less social cohesion. These children scored significantly lower (better) on a scale measuring their psychological stress experience.

We consider the measures included in this study to be indicators of positive health because they have internal validity in both positive and negative valences. For example, measures of child behavior (e.g., using the Child Behavior Checklist – CBCL), which is frequently used in environmental epidemiology research, is able to detect behavior problems but not well-equipped to discern behavior within the normal range (28). The positive health scales included in this study were designed to be able to parse indicators in the positive, non-clinical range. It is critically important to have valid measures in the positive valence, particularly when trying to identify environmental factors that promote child health beyond the prevention of disease or disorder. These indicators have not been widely used in children's environmental health research and provide an opportunity to identify points for intervention. Our use of the PROMIS positive health scales attempt to address this gap. Further, the assessment of positive health in longitudinal studies across childhood and adolescence is of particular importance because it allows for the identification of potential sensitive periods when environmental exposures, social interactions or biophysical transitions may have disproportionate effects.

Previously, our group examined neighborhood quality in relation to childhood mood disorders and found that stressed neighborhood quality across middle childhood is associated with an increase in maternally-reported symptoms of depression in children at age 9-12 years (28). In this follow-up work, we wanted to know whether the same indicators of neighborhood quality were associated with positive health outcomes in children as they age (median age in this study: 16 years).

Although not significant, our observed inverse relationship between perceived NQ (stressed versus non-stressed NQ indicator variables for overall, safety and order) and our positive health outcome, life satisfaction, is consistent with previous studies in both adults (18, 19) and adolescents (23), which reported higher life satisfaction with greater perceived NQ using various indicators of NQ. To our knowledge, our study is one of the few to evaluate the relationship between perceived neighborhood quality and children's general health using a positively valenced robust and dimensional measure of overall health that accounts for physical, mental and social components. Though work on NQ and HRQoL exists (15, 31), the studies often focus on physical or mental health outcomes, treat the absence of health problems as the presence of well-being, and evaluate neighborhood deprivation derived from administrative data rather than quality indicators from proxy/self-report. However, our non-significant findings of lower global health reported in stressed NQ groups compared to non-stressed groups (for overall NQ, safety and order) is consistent with previous work reporting associations between higher perceived neighborhood quality and greater HRQoL (32–34). In addition, our findings of greater stress and sleep disturbance in all stressed NQ groups compared to non-stressed groups is consistent with numerous studies that have identified the detrimental effect of poor perceived NQ on both of these outcomes (20, 35–39). Highlighting the importance of these relationships, both poor sleep and stress have been indicated as potential mediators in the pathway between NQ and negative health outcomes (20, 37).

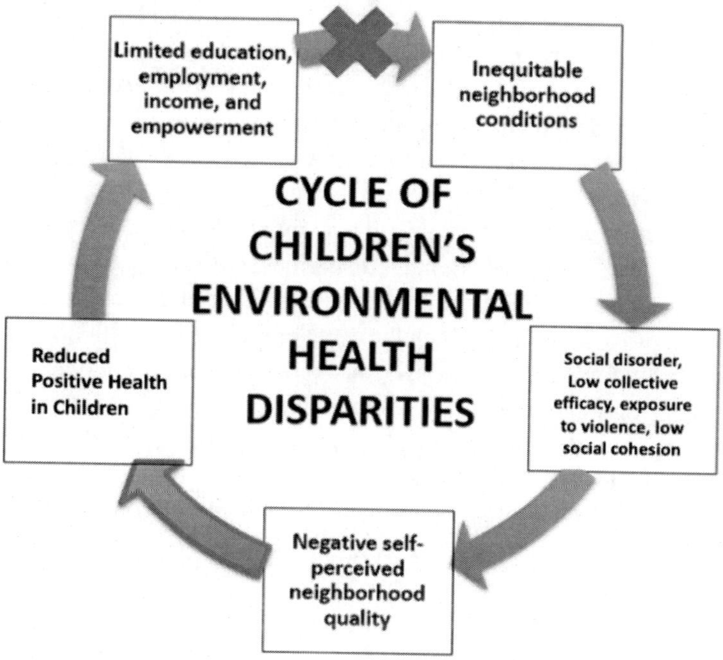

Figure 3. Breaking the Cycle of Environmental Health Disparities related to neighborhood quality and children's positive health.

In our study, the only significant finding with the parent proxy of positive health was between the NQ indicator of higher perceived social cohesion and psychological stress. Social cohesion is an important component of neighborhood quality that represents strong social ties within a community and a sense of neighborhood support and connectedness. Numerous studies have found associations between greater perceived social cohesion (including related concepts such as neighborhood social capital and social efficacy) and better self-reported health in both adults (40–44), adolescents (45) and children (46). Relevant to our study, some findings have indicated this relationship may be stronger in urban areas compared to rural (41). Different pathways between neighborhood social cohesion and health have been hypothesized. One theory suggests social cohesion develops a social environment with fewer risks, while others pose that its development of safety nets and acquisition of community resources is what links it to better health

(47). In terms of stress, to our knowledge, just one study has evaluated the relationship between perceived neighborhood social cohesion and this health outcome. In a study of single mothers from the US, the relationship between neighborhood disorder and maternal stress was mediated by perceived social capital (42). Within a smaller sub-population, we observed significant associations between maternally reported overall NQ and the safety NQ scale and child self-reported Global Health. These findings are in the same direction as the analyses conducted within the larger sample with parent proxy measures.

This study was conducted in the context of the Break the Cycle of Children's Environmental Health Disparities (BTC) program, a research program that allows students to engage with topics in children's environmental health and propose ways in which the cycle of children's health disparities can be broken. We expanded on a previous BTC study exploring neighborhood quality and children's depressive symptoms (28) to evaluate the degree to which neighborhood quality may also affect positive health outcomes in children. As shown in Figure 3, we have identified a point of intervention that we believe can reduce disproportionate differences in youth wellbeing. By studying various aspects of longitudinally assessed neighborhood characteristics and children's positive health, we are able to identify a specific aspect of neighborhood quality that may be especially influential: social cohesion. Our analysis highlights that, compared to neighborhood safety and social order, increased social cohesion may have a strong impact on children's positive health indices, including psychological stress and sleep. Therefore, initiatives designed to improve community-based social cohesiveness may provide opportunities to "break the cycle" of children's health disparities, as it relates to the quality of a child's neighborhood environment.

Strengths and limitations

Our study has a number of strengths. First, neighborhood quality was assessed prospectively and longitudinally (at child ages 5, 7, 9 and 11 years), which is critical as neighborhood quality may be difficult to recall retrospectively. The measures of NQ were prior to our assessment of positive health, an outcome that has not yet been well-studied among children or adolescents. By including this measure in our longitudinal cohort study, we can begin to understand factors that promote and predict positive health outcomes among children and adolescents. One notable limitation of our study was that we relied primarily on maternal reports of child positive health, which may be significantly different from child self-report, particularly among older children. However, in the subset of adolescents for whom we have both maternal proxy and child self-report, these differences were not significant. Both maternal proxy and child self-reported positive health have been nationally normed, allowing us to compare our population to a normative sample. One limitation of our research is that the neighborhood quality assessed in the study was based on the mother's perception. It is possible that as children grow older, they are more conscious about the attributes – both positive and negative – of their own neighborhood. As the child is most likely doing different things in the neighborhood than the mother, the maternal perceived NQ might be slightly different than how the child perceived and values the neighborhood. Another limitation is that our assessment of NQ trajectory ended at child age 11 years and the outcomes reported here were assessed much later (median age: 16 years). There are likely other factors – both precision variables and potential confounders – that we did not measure or consider that might account for some of the variation in positive health outcomes. Because of the wide age range of the positive health measures, we were not able to focus on potentially sensitive developmental windows for positive health (e.g., puberty, transition to high school, college/work force). Future work, potentially within the context of the ECHO consortium may be able to address some of these questions.

Conclusion

In our study, we observed a general trend of better reported child and adolescent health with higher perceived neighborhood quality. Specifically, we observed a significant association between neighborhood social cohesion and psychological stress experience (as reported by the mothers) and between overall neighborhood quality and neighborhood safety and Global Health (as self-reported by the child). These under-recognized relationships suggest that initiatives designed to break the cycle of childrens' environmental health disparities may be most impactful at improving child positive health indicators by focusing on fostering neighborhood social cohesiveness and the overall safety of neighborhoods.

References

[1] VanderWeele TJ, Chen Y, Long K, Kim ES, Trudel-Fitzgerald C, Kubzansky LD. Positive epidemiology? Epidemiology 2020;31(2):189–93.

[2] Health-Related Quality of Life and Well-Being. URL: https://www.healthypeople.gov/2020/topics-objectives/topic/health-related-quality-of-life-well-being.

[3] Diener E, Seligman MEP. Beyond money: toward an economy of well-being. Psychol Sci Public Interest 2004;5(1):1–31.

[4] Cohen R, Bavishi C, Rozanski A. Purpose in life and its relationship to all-cause mortality and cardiovascular events: a meta-analysis. Psychosom Med 2016;78(2):122–33.

[5] Martín-María N, Miret M, Caballero FF, Rico-Uribe LA, Steptoe A, Chatterji S, et al. The impact of subjective well-being on mortality: a meta-analysis of longitudinal studies in the general population. Psychosom Med 2017;79(5):565–75.

[6] Pressman SD, Cohen S. Does positive affect influence health? Psychol Bull 2005;131(6):925–71.

[7] Ryff CD, Dienberg Love G, Urry HL, Muller D, Rosenkranz MA, Friedman EM, et al. Psychological well-being and ill-being: do they have distincet or mirrored biological correlates? Psychother Psychosom 2006;75(2):85–95.

[8] Forrest CB, Blackwell CK, Camargo CA Jr. Advancing the science of children's positive health in the National Institutes of Health Environmental Influences on Child Health Outcomes (ECHO) Research Program. J Pediatr 2018;196:298–300.

[9] Rollings KA, Wells NM, Evans GW. Measuring physical neighborhood quality related to health. Behav Sci 2015;5(2):190–202.

[10] Diez Roux AV, Mair C. Neighborhoods and health. Ann NY Acad Sci 2010;1186:125–45.

[11] Renalds A, Smith TH, Hale PJ. A systematic review of built environment and health. Fam Commun Health 2010;33(1):68–78.

[12] Weden MM, Carpiano RM, Robert SA. Subjective and objective neighborhood characteristics and adult health. Soc Sci Med 2008;66(6):1256–70.

[13] Wen M, Hawkley LC, Cacioppo JT. Objective and perceived neighborhood environment, individual SES and psychosocial factors, and self-rated health: An analysis of older adults in Cook County, Illinois. Soc Sci Med 2006;63(1):2575–90. URL: http://dx.doi.org/10.1016/j.socscimed.2006.06.025.

[14] Kipke MD, Iverson E, Moore D, Booker C, Ruelas V, Peters AL, et al. Food and park environments: neighborhood-level risks for childhood obesity in east Los Angeles. J Adolesc Health 2007;40(4):325–33.

[15] Leventhal T, Brooks-Gunn J. The neighborhoods they live in: the effects of neighborhood residence on child and adolescent outcomes. Psychol Bull 2000;126(2):309–37.

[16] Ding D, Sallis JF, Kerr J, Lee S, Rosenberg DE. Neighborhood environment and physical activity among youth a review. Am J Prev Med 2011;41(4):442–55.

[17] Schaefer-McDaniel N. Neighborhood stressors, perceived neighborhood quality, and child mental health in New York City. Health Place 2009;15(1):148–55.

[18] Stokes JE. Trajectories of perceived neighborhood quality across the life course: Sociodemographic determinants and implications for well-being. Soc Sci Res 2019;79:181–93.

[19] Ma J, Dong G, Chen Y, Zhang W. Does satisfactory neighbourhood environment lead to a satisfying life? An investigation of the association between neighbourhood environment and life satisfaction in Beijing. Cities 2018;74:229–39. URL: http://dx.doi.org/10.1016/j.cities.2017.12.008.

[20] Hale L, Hill TD, Friedman E, Nieto FJ, Galvao LW, Engelman CD, et al. Perceived neighborhood quality, sleep quality, and health status: evidence from the Survey of the Health of Wisconsin. Soc Sci Med 2013;79:16–22.

[21] Kamimura A, Christensen N, Prevedel JA, Tabler J, Hamilton BJ, Ashby J, et al. Quality of life among free clinic patients associated with somatic symptoms, depression, and perceived neighborhood environment. J Commun Health 2014;39(3):524–30.

[22] Zhang F, Li D. Multiple linear regression-structural equation modeling based development of the integrated model of perceived neighborhood environment and quality of life of community-dwelling older adults: A cross-sectional study in Nanjing, China. International J Environ Res Public Health 2019;16:4933. URL: http://dx.doi.org/10.3390/ijerph16244933.

[23] Valois RF, Kerr JC, Carey MP, Brown LK, Romer D, DiClemente RJ, et al. Neighborhood stress and life satisfaction: is there a relationship for African American adolescents? Appl Res Qual Life 2020;15(1):273–96.

[24] Whyatt RM, Camann DE, Kinney PL, Reyes A, Ramirez J, Dietrich J, et al. Residential pesticide use during pregnancy among a cohort of urban minority women. Environ Health Perspect 2002;110:507–14. URL: http://dx.doi.org/10.1289/ehp.02110507.

[25] Kim SY, Nair R, Knight GP, Roosa MW, Updegraff KA. Measurement equivalence of neighborhood quality measures for european american and mexican american familes. J Commun Psychol 2008;37(1):1–20.

[26] Sampson RJ. Neighborhoods and violent crime: A multilevel study of collective efficacy. Science. 1997;277:918–24. URL: http://dx.doi.org/10.1126/science.277.5328.918.

[27] Sampson RJ, Raudenbush SW. Systematic social observation of public spaces: a new look at disorder in the urban neighborhoods. Social observation of public spaces: A new look at disorder in urban neighborhoods. Am J Sociol 1999;105(3):603–51.

[28] Bs DT, Margolis A, Pagliaccio D, Mha GW, Mph RKW. Self-perceived neighborhood quality and children's depression symptoms in a gentrifying Northern Manhattan. Int J Child Health Hum Dev 2019;12:413–24.

[29] Hays RD, Bjorner JB, Revicki DA, Spritzer KL, Cella D. Development of physical and mental health summary scores from the patient-reported outcomes measurement information system (PROMIS) global items. Qual Life Res 2009;18(7):873–80.

[30] Reeve BB, Hays RD, Bjorner JB, Cook KF, Crane PK, Teresi JA, et al. Psychometric evaluation and calibration of health-related quality of life item banks:

plans for the Patient-Reported Outcomes Measurement Information System (PROMIS). Med Care 2007;45(5 Suppl 1):S22–31.
[31] van Vuuren CL, Reijneveld SA, van der Wal MF, Verhoeff AP. Neighborhood socioeconomic deprivation characteristics in child (0–18 years) health studies: A review. Health Place 2014;29:34–42.
[32] Toma A, Hamer M, Shankar A. Associations between neighborhood perceptions and mental well-being among older adults. Health Place 2015;34:46–53.
[33] Robinette JW, Charles ST, Mogle JA, Almeida DM. Neighborhood cohesion and daily well-being: results from a diary study. Soc Sci Med 2013;96:174–82.
[34] Snedker KA, Hooven C. Neighborhood perceptions and emotional well-being in young adulthood. J Child Adolesc Psychiatr Nurs 2013;26(1):62–73.
[35] Henderson H, Child S, Moore S, Moore JB, Kaczynski AT. The influence of neighborhood aesthetics, safety, and social cohesion on perceived stress in disadvantaged communities. Am J Community Psychol 2016;58(1-2):80–8.
[36] Lamis DA, Wilson CK, Tarantino N, Lansford JE, Kaslow NJ. Neighborhood disorder, spiritual well-being, and parenting stress in African American women. J Fam Psychol 2014;28(6):769–78.
[37] Giurgescu C, Misra DP, Sealy-Jefferson S, Caldwell CH, Templin TN, Slaughter-Acey JC, et al. The impact of neighborhood quality, perceived stress, and social support on depressive symptoms during pregnancy in African American women. Soc Sci Med 2015;130:172–80.
[38] Hill TD, Burdette AM, Hale L. Neighborhood disorder, sleep quality, and psychological distress: testing a model of structural amplification. Health Place 2009;15(4):1006–13.
[39] Hill TD, Trinh HN, Wen M, Hale L. Perceived neighborhood safety and sleep quality: a global analysis of six countries. Sleep Med 2016;18:56–60.
[40] Mohnen SM, Völker B, Flap H, Subramanian SV. The influence of social capital on individual health: is it the neighbourhood or the network? Soc Indic Res 2015;121:195-214. URL: https://link.springer.com/article/10.1007%252Fs11205-014-0632-8.
[41] Mohnen SM, Groenewegen PP, Völker B, Flap H. Neighborhood social capital and individual health. Soc Sci Med 2011;72(5):660–7.
[42] Zhang S, Eamon MK, Zhan M. Neighborhood disorder, perceptions of neighborhood social capital, and maternal stress: Exploration of a mediating mechanism. J Commun Psychol 2015;43(3):278–95.
[43] Browning CR, Cagney KA. Neighborhood structural disadvantage, collective efficacy, and self-rated physical health in an urban setting. J Health Soc Behav 2002;43(4):383–99.
[44] Rios R, Aiken LS, Zautra AJ. Neighborhood contexts and the mediating role of neighborhood social cohesion on health and psychological distress among Hispanic and non-Hispanic residents. Ann Behav Med 2012;43(1):50–61.
[45] Abada T, Hou F, Ram B. Racially mixed neighborhoods, perceived neighborhood social cohesion, and adolescent health in Canada. Soc Sci Med 2007;65(10):2004–17.

[46] Curtis LJLJ, Dooley MDMD, Phipps SASA. Child well-being and neighbourhood quality: Evidence from the Canadian National Longitudinal Survey of Children and Youth. Soc Sci Med 2004;58(10):1917–27.

[47] Drukker M, Buka SL, Kaplan C, McKenzie K, Van Os J. Social capital and young adolescents' perceived health in different sociocultural settings. Soc Sci Med 2005;61:185–98. URL: http://dx.doi.org/10.1016/j.socscimed.2004.11.041.

Chapter 9

A grief group for today's teens: Using human-centered design to develop an evidence-based intervention for teens that have lost a parent

Julia Chavez[1,*], BA, Jessica Cheng[1], BA, Amelie Liu[2], HSD, Alexis Hansen[3], SWLC, Jesse Boring[3], PhD, Irwin Sandler[5,6], PhD and Dana Suskind[7], MD

[1]Pritzker School of Medicine, University of Chicago, Chicago, Illinois, United States of America
[2]University of Chicago Laboratory Schools, University of Chicago, Chicago, Illinois, United States of America
[3]Crown Family School of Social Work, Policy, and Practice, University of Chicago, Chicago, Illinois, United States of America
[4]Psychology and Human Services Department, SUNY Broome Community College, Binghamton, New York, United States of America
[5]REACH Institute, Arizona State University, Tempe, Arizona, United States of America
[6]Department of Psychology, Arizona State University, Tempe, Arizona, United States of America
[7]Department of Surgery, University of Chicago Medicine, Chicago, Illinois, United States of America

Abstract

Parent loss during childhood is a profoundly stressful life event affecting one in 25 individuals in the United States. Early parent loss places children at risk for both short- and long-term negative health and life outcomes, including mental health issues (e.g., depression, anxiety, post

[*] *Correspondence:* Julia Chavez, BA, Medical Student, Pritzker School of Medicine, University of Chicago. Email: juliachavez@mac.com.

traumatic stress disorder) and lower academic success. Given the potential negative sequelae across the lifespan, timely intervention is critical. In this study, we used human-centered design (HCD) to develop an evidence-based intervention for teens who have lost a parent, using the Family Bereavement Program (FBP) as a model. A new peer-led delivery model was introduced to the curriculum, as well as the incorporation of technology and mindfulness strategies. We recruited researchers and members of the target population to provide feedback on the curriculum in focus groups. The results of focus group testing indicated that there are theory-practice gaps within post-bereavement interventions that can be identified and redressed through human-centered design framework. The focus group feedback provided preliminary support for the peer-led curriculum for parentally-bereaved teens as well as suggestions for adaptation and modifications. Future work will be centered around further refining the model ensuring fidelity and scalability of the intervention.

Introduction

Parent loss during childhood is a profoundly stressful life event affecting one in 25 individuals in the United States (1, 2). Early parent loss places children at risk for both short- and long-term negative health and life outcomes, including mental health issues (e.g., depression, anxiety, post traumatic stress disorder) and lower academic success (3–5). Race and socioeconomic status are associated with increased prevalence and earlier timing of parent loss, contributing to social and health inequities (1, 6). The COVID-19 pandemic led to increased rates of parent loss in the United States, raising concerns that the pandemic is exacerbating pre-existing social disparities (7). Researchers found the risk of loss was 1.1 to 4.5 times higher in minority groups compared with White children during the pandemic (7). Given the potential negative sequelae across the lifespan, timely evidence-based intervention focused on children at greatest risk is critical.

However, few evidence-based services are available to children grieving the death of a parent. One exception is the Family Bereavement Program (FBP), the most extensively researched intervention for parentally-bereaved children (8). The FBP is a 12-week skill-based group curriculum targeting mediating factors for mental health and resilience, such as positive coping, threat appraisals, adaptive emotional expression, and caregiver-child relationship quality. Results from a randomized control trial demonstrated that the FBP improved mental health and coping measures and that these effects persisted for up to 15 years after the end of the program (9, 10). The caregiver portion of the FBP curriculum has continued to be updated, however, the most recent version of the child and adolescent module is from 1995.

In the last 25 years, personal digital devices and technology have become ubiquitous and over 95% of teenagers, across socioeconomic backgrounds, have access to a smartphone (11). Online peer-to-peer support is increasingly gaining traction as a way to promote mental and physical wellbeing. It provides a helpful and supportive environment that allows individuals facing an isolating condition (e.g., parental bereavement) to feel connected to others going through similar experiences (12, 13). Furthermore, growing recognition of the consequences of trauma exposure has led to calls for the incorporation of trauma-informed care and mindfulness in psychosocial interventions (14, 15).

In this chapter, we will use human-centered design (HCD) to update the FBP in order to develop a program that is accessible and engaging to teens today. By collaborating with researchers, practitioners, and parentally-bereaved adolescents, we aim to develop a program that utilizes the most current and evidence-supported modalities, while using an approach that is feasible for practitioners and engaging to teens.

Our study

In adapting the FBP curriculum, we employed HCD, a design method that stems from the idea that interventions are more effective when they are developed with— not just for—the people who will ultimately use the intervention. Collaborating with key stakeholders throughout the design process helps to increase intervention uptake by ensuring that the intervention is structured to meet the community's and users' needs rather than those perceived by the research team, and mitigate the "research-practice gap" (16, 17).

The adaptation of the intervention occurred in three phases. In Phase 1, the FBP curriculum was identified as a framework and was adapted to an initial protype. We maintained the core components of promoting evidence-based coping skills from the FBP curriculum and made the following key adaptations: the development of a peer-led adult-supported curriculum delivery model and the addition of mindfulness practice. In Phase 2, subject-matter experts – researchers and practitioners – provided feedback on the adapted program. In Phase 3, we conducted focus groups with members of the target population. Consistent with the principles of HCD, all phases of the development process occurred with a parentally-bereaved adolescent at the center of the decision-making process.

Phase 1: Problem identification and initial prototype

The research team met with six local Chicago-area grief centers and evaluated the various options employed at each center. The major finding was that many grief centers conduct unstructured, process-based groups in which the focus is on processing the emotional significance of the loss, in part because evidence-based resources were difficult to access. The Family Bereavement Program emerged as the most extensively researched support program for families in which one parent has died, and thus was selected as the foundation of the adaptation (18).

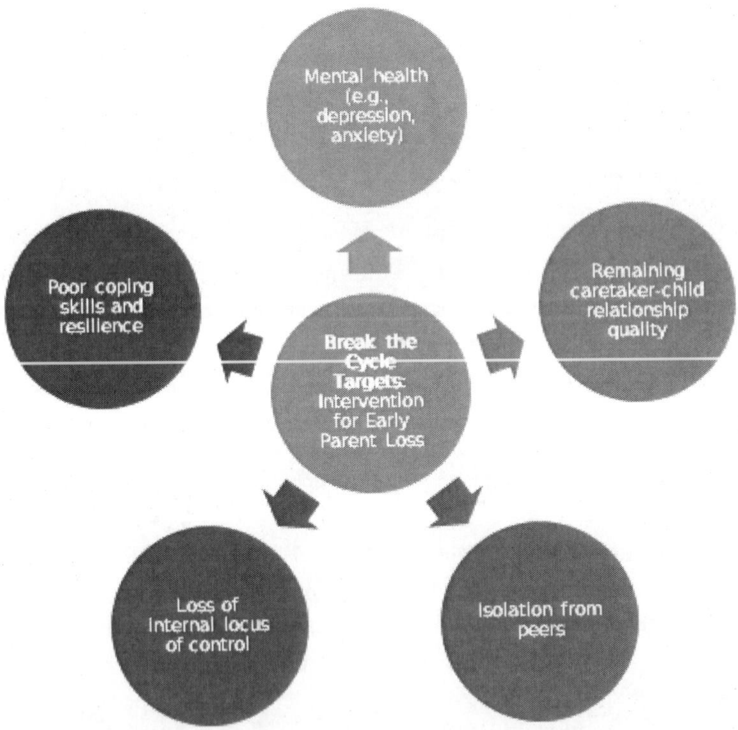

Figure 1. The cycle of early parent loss and the targets for breaking the cycle.

The FBP is a skills-based program designed to promote resilience through modification of the variables that affect the mental health of bereaved children (see Figure 1: the cycle of early parent loss) (19). Over the course of 12 sessions, the program promotes known protective factors (positive coping, coping efficacy, adaptive control beliefs, adaptive emotional expression, caregiver-child relationship) while reducing known risk factors (negative esteem and threat appraisals) During each session, participants learn a new coping skill each week (i.e., identifying and challenging cognitive distortions, healthy emotional boundaries, problem-solving and communication, etc.) and discuss strategies to use and apply the skills outside the group meetings.

The initial adaptation of the FBP was guided by the following principles, which were identified through a collaborative process with both subject-matter experts and members of the target population:

1. *Addition of mindfulness.* Mindfulness is the practice of awareness and nonjudgmental acceptance of one's moment-to-moment experience. We decided to add mindfulness to the program due to its evidence-based benefits in addressing early childhood trauma by enhancing emotional regulation, positive coping skills, and resilience (15, 20, 21). Mindfulness is introduced to participants during the first lesson and is subsequently reinforced through a short practice at the end of every lesson.
2. *Peer-led programming:* The original program is co-led by two trained adult leaders. However, the adapted program is designed to be co-led by a teen leader (a parentally-bereaved adolescent) and an adult supervisor. We found early evidence of support for the acceptability and efficacy of peer-led mental health curriculums (22–24). Furthermore, the new design employs the fundamental framework of human-centered design, where the stakeholders and leaders include the end-users.
3. *Opportunities to increase accessibility and youth engagement:* To make the curriculum more engaging to participants, we made two major changes. First, the adapted curriculum was framed as a community building experience rather than a school classroom experience. For example, the language throughout the program was also modified to be less clinical and more youthful (a review session originally titled "Relapse Prevention" was re-titled "Bring It!"; the assigned "homework" was renamed "personal practice"). Second, interactive technologies were integrated throughout the curriculum.

For example, worksheets were replaced with online quizzes (PollEv.com and Kahoot!).

4. *Modified audience to target adolescents only:* Whereas the original FBP was designed for both the bereaved child and their caregiver, in the adapted program, the adolescent module was made independent from the caregiver module. Some aspects of the adapted program still address the caregiver-child relationship, but to a lesser extent than in the original program.
5. *Condensed program for more flexibility in delivery:* The program was shortened from twelve 2-hour sessions to ten 1-hour sessions in order to allow for more flexibility in implementation (e.g., it is more feasible to implement the curriculum as an after-school program if the time commitment is just one hour per week). Also, the program was adapted from an in-person model to a virtual setting through the use of Zoom video-conferencing. This change was initially made to accommodate social distancing restrictions of the coronavirus pandemic. However, even without social distancing restrictions, a virtual delivery also allows for increased flexibility in delivering the program and increased accesibility.

Importantly, the core components of the FBP were preserved. The specific coping skills taught over the course of the program were taught using a similar framework. The developer of the original FBP was consulted throughout the process to ensure that the adaptation maintained fidelity to the principles underlying the original FBP.

Phase 2: Subject-matter expert feedback and responsive iteration

We recruited researchers and practitioners with backgrounds in the following areas: trauma-informed care, mindfulness, grief group facilitation, curriculum development, grief and coping, group dynamics and child/adolescent psychiatry. We conducted semi-structured interviews with subject-matter experts (15 experts, 34 interviews). Interviews began with a review of the curriculum goals and an example lesson plan; experts were encouraged to provide feedback on the curriculum adaptations. Interviews closed with questions specific to their field(s) of expertise.

Following each interview, the research team reviewed all comments, suggestions, and unanswered questions that arose during the interview. Suggested changes were either implemented, modified, or otherwise addressed (e.g., with an explanation for why no change was made). Questions or points of discussion were included in plans for future expert meetings or focus groups.

Phase 3: Target population feedback and responsive iteration

Members of the target population were recruited to provide feedback in focus groups with parent permission. Potential participants were recruited through an announcement to an online community for teens that have lost a parent (Surviving life after a parent dies, @slapdstories). Interested members and their parent/guardian then discussed involvment with the research team. Ultimately, nine adolescents were included in the focus groups. Participants were ages 14-18 years and had experienced the death of a parent between 1-7 years prior.

We conducted two focus groups with parentally-bereaved adolescents (nine teens, 12 focus group sessions). Focus group A (N = 4) participated in an accelerated version of the full curriculum, meeting 10 times over the course of two weeks. The group ran through every lesson in the curriculum. Each lesson was followed by a 20-minute feedback session. Focus group B (N = 5) provided targeted feedback across two sessions. During these sessions, they provided feedback in two ways. They either directly discussed quesstions that had come up during prior feedback sessions or they would test out two variations of an activity and then provide feedback. The research team met after every focus group session to review all comments and suggestions, modifying the lessons or activities as appropriate.

The intervention, after following feedback and responsive iteration throughout phases 1-3, is described below.

The adapted program consists of ten one-hour sessions that each follows the same structure: lesson title and theme, check-in, experiential activity and discussion, mindfulness, check-out (25). The coping skills covered in each session are detailed in Table 1. Selected slides from lesson 6 are shown in Figure 2 to illustrate the structure of each lesson.

Each session begins with “Welcome Bback!” during which the “teen leader” (TL) reviews the day’s plan and processes participants’ experiences with their personal practice from the week before. The TL then leads the “activity” and “discussion” portion of the session in which an activity is used to introduce a coping skill and the group then discusses the activity. As the session comess to a close, the “adult support” (AS) leads a mindfulness exercise. Finally, each session concludes with the “check out” in which participants recap the takeaways for the week and discuss a personal practice assignment related to the coping skill they learned during that session.

Table 1. Lesson titles and skills

Wk	Meeting title	Skills or coping strategies
1	Navigating Loss, Finding My People	Introduction to mindfulness Foster relationships with peers
2	Inside Out	Communicating positive messages at home Focusing on positives
3	Utility of Thoughts	Identifying andmonitoring thoughts. Replacing harmful thoughts with hopeful thoughts
4	Being Seen, Being Heard, Being Supported	Seeking emotional support from parents/caregiver by: – Identifying barriers to good communication – Using I-Messages
5	Relax and Reflect	Reinforcing mindfulness practice Practice gratitude and reflection Deepen relationships with peers through vulnerability
6	Carrying the World on Your Shoulders	Distinguishing between responsibilities that do and don’t belong to a teen
7	Be Your Own Superhero	Problem solving ‘not your job scenarios’
8	Piece of My Heart	Renegotiating relationship with parent who passed away
9	Bring It!	Review of skills and discussions
10	Celebrating Us	Celebrating accomplishments

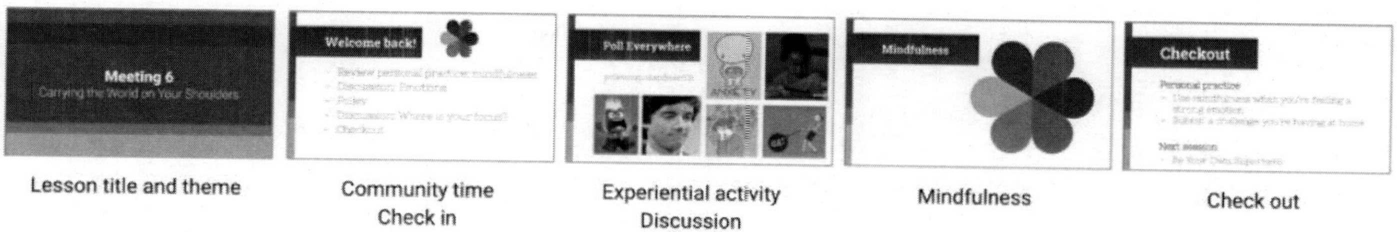

Figure 2. Recurring structure.

Our findings

Most experts endorsed the use of a peer-led delivery model, noting that peer-to-peer mentoring is very effective, especially with a younger population. Experts also highlighted the unique ability of a peer-facilitator to allow for behavioral modeling and to enhance coping efficacy. Experts also noted that peer-led interventions are compelling due to their relatively lower resource requirement and their ability to leverage social influence and peer attachment, which are particularly important during the teen years.

However, some experts also noted the importance of adult supervision to ensure the safety and efficacy of the model. One expert commented: "I would want someone with at least a master's level, at least. You don't want that teen who's leading the group holding [the] complexity [of traumatic grief]. … I would build in some kind of supervision for the leaders, and that supervision can be focused on what's coming up in the group and problem solving around that if need be."

In response to feedback, a special effort was made to ensure that the teen and adult leaders were more effectively integrated into the group. To do this, the role of the adult leader was expanded and more clearly defined. The primary purpose of the trained therapist remained to ensure psychological and emotional safety during the sessions by troubleshooting more advanced issues, such as concerns with group dynamics or cases in which a participant would benefit from a higher level of support (e.g., therapy).. However, the adult leader was also given the responsibility of addressing more advanced topics, such as the distinction between sadness and depression, as appropriate. The aim was to make the roles of the teen and adult leaders distinct and complementary. The title was changed from "adult supervisor" to "adult support" to reflect this modification.

Teen feedback

The peer-led model was positively received by the teens in the focus groups. One participant stated: "I have gone to support groups where we share with an adult and we don't exactly think the same as them, so it was nice to hear comments from someone that is at our level." Another said: "It's just nice to know that you're not alone…. Other people are experiencing something similar to you, and it just helps to know that other people are going through it and you [too] will get through it."

Coping skills

Expert feedback

Experts endorsed the importance of the coping skills being taught, a finding which reinforced the strength of the original program on which this adaptation was based. Experts commented that teens would respond well to sophisticated explanations. As a result of this feedback, the importance of coping skills was discussed in the context of neuroplasticity. Participants were told that practicing the strategies for emotional identification and expression would reinforce different behavioral and thus neural patterns. Experts also suggested discussing the physical aspects of emotion and the purpose of emotions from an evolutionary perspective during the discussions about emotional awareness and mindfulness; this too was added to the lesson.

Teen feedback

In general, the coping skill lessons were very well received by the participants. The changes suggested by the experts helped to enhance the lessons. The discussion about neuroplasticity resonated strongly with participants. As stated above, participants were told that practicing the strategies from the would reinforce different behavioral and thus neural patterns. One participant put it this way: "The material is helpful for *re-wiring* your brain for more positive thinking." The discussion about neuroplasticity led to a discussion about how each time one uses one of the more adaptive coping skills helps to make that strategy even easier to implement in the future, and in turn, this idea helped to reinforce the importance of personal practice between the sessions. In addition, teens responded well to the discussion about the physical aspect and evolutionary purpose of emotions. They noted that this was a new perspective for them, and it helped them better understand the utility of mindfulness in coping with grief.

Participants reported that it was most helpful when the lesson on a coping skill was followed by a discussion about specific contexts in which the skill would be helpful. For example, after the lesson on using "I" messages to improve communication, participants were asked to consider an example in the past week when this communication strategy would have improved an interaction. One participant commented "I knew about "I" messages already but an a-ha moment for me was when [the teen leader] asked when I could have used it and I realized maybe this could've gone better if I had tried this instead."

One major change was made to the lesson about emotion recognition as a result of teen feedback. Initially, the lessons about various emotions (e.g., anger, guilt, sadness, etc) were spread across multiple sessions. During the pilot testing, the first session, which focused on the emotion 'anger,' was poorly received. The participants generally felt that the session did not resonate with them and none of the learning objectives were met. In response to this, all the lessons on emotion recognition and coping were collapsed into a single session. This version performed much better in pilot testing. It was much better received by the teens who now reported finding the session very helpful and illuminating. They reported that it helped them see their emotional experience from a different perspective. Participants were able to reflect on the specific feelings they were experiencing, rather than generically sharing that they felt "badly." One participant commented on the realization that it is easier to cope with feeling both sad and angry once you have labeled those as distinct feelings: "I think if you bundle [negative emotions] all together, it can be like really overwhelming, and it can just be like a lot all at once, but instead if you separate them you can deal with them separately."

Teen feedback also revealed that the sessions with clearer structure and skill-focus were better received than those that were more fluid. This finding contradicted our original hypothesis. In fact, we had originally de-emphasized "home practice" in the initial prototype so that the program did not involve "homework," but then during the teen feedback sessions, we found that the remaining elements of home practice consistently received positive feedback from participants. In response to this feedback, we re-introduced some structure into the lessons. Key takeaways from each lesson were discussed during the beginning and end of each lesson. Also, home practice – rebranded as "personal practice" – was re-emphasized throughout the program. Each week, participants were encouraged to discuss real-world examples of when a given skill would be – or could have been – helpful. The renewed emphasis on the importance of practicing skills outside of the lessons represented a return to one of the core components of the original FBP that had been de-emphasized during phase 1. While it is possible that reducing the emphasis of "homework" could have helped to make the adapted program more engaging, responsive iteration revealed that structure and skill reinforcement actually enhanced the participant experience. This was an especially important finding given that home practice is regarded as one of the key elements of the FBP which drives the efficacy of the program.

Mindfulness

Mindfulness is the practice of awareness and acceptance of one's moment-to-moment experience without judgment (15, 21). Experts supported the incorporation of mindfulness practice at the end of each lesson. Participants began with a 30 second practice and the time increased over the course of the ten sessions.

Expert feedback

Experts supported the incorporation of mindfulness practice as a thread throughout the program rather than the focus of a single lesson. When mindfulness is first introduced, the teen leader provides a personal example of success with mindfulness. Experts supported this anecdote as an important way to encourage skeptical participants to try this new skill with an open mind. Following the feedback of multiple experts, a metaphor illustrating the value of mindfulness was added to the first lesson in which mindfulness is introduced.

Teen feedback

One surprising finding was the extent to which the mindfulness resonated with participants. During one session, the session closed with a game instead of mindfulness practice and the participant feedback suggested we add mindfulness practice back in. During the first lesson, when mindfulness was introduced, the TL encouraged participants to keep an open mind. She commented that she too was initially unsure about the utility of mindfulness for her personally, but that she come to enjoy it and find it beneficial. It is possible that these comments helped to ease potential skepticism from participants.

Discussion

The results of phase 3 focus group testing indicated that there are theory-practice gaps within post-bereavement interventions that can be identified and redressed through a human-centered design framework. The responsive iterative process was important to ensure the changes made to the curriculum were structured to meet both the recommendations of researchers and the needs of parentally-bereaved teens. Two elements of the curriculum which demonstrated the utility of responsive iteration are described below.

First, the lessons on emotion recognition and coping benefitted greatly from consultation with both experts and teens. Initially, this skill was taught longitudinally across several sessions, each addressing a single emotion. Feedback from experts was considered and integrated. However, it was not until the lessons on emotion recognition and coping were collapsed into a single session that the lesson was effective. Whereas teens initially stated that the lesson did not resonate with them, they later reported that it was one of their favorite sessions. This modification also had the unintended benefit of reinforcing the importance of the ability to distinguish between similar but different emotions, an important emotion regulation skill called "emotional granulation." The efficacy of the emotion recognition lessons were greatly enhanced by the iterative HCD process.

Second, the novel peer-led delivery model was consistently praised by teens but was generally met with skepticism from experts. Thus finding a feasible way to implement the peer-led model was a priority during the adaptation process and it was one that also benefitted from HCD. While teens commented on the importance of learning from a peer they can relate to, experts initially raised concerns about the ability of the teen leader to navigate the complexity of grief in other teens. Throughout the expert feedback process, the responsibilities of the adult leader were expanded and more clearly defined in order to allow for a safe and supportive environment with close supervision while also keeping the program centered on the teen participants. Initial experiences with the program suggest that the use of an "adult support" as a co-leader has the potential to effectively address expert concerns. However, it will be critical to develop an effective facilitator-training process in the future.

This study provides preliminary support for the peer-led curriculum for parentally-bereaved teens. We hope that early and accessible intervention will break the cycle of disparities, particularly for children at greatest risk for early parent loss and negative health consequences that were exacerbated by the pandemic. Future work will involve the addition of a training program for the teen and adult co-facilitators to ensure the program can be replicated with fidelity as well as pilot testing to ensure feasibility and scalability he eventual goal will be to test the curriculum in randomized controlled trials to assess the efficacy of the program in promoting adaptive coping in adolescents experiencing parental loss.

Acknowledgments

This work was supported by the University of Chicago Bucksbaum Institute for Clinical Excellence and Break the Cycle of Children's Environmental Health Disparities.

References

[1] Sherer Z. Parental mortality is linked to a variety of socio-economic and demographic factors. URL: https://www.census.gov/library/stories/2019/05/when-do-we-lose-our-parents.html.

[2] Burns M, Griese B, King S, Tami A. Childhood bereavement: Understanding prevalence and related adversity in the United States. Am J Orthopsychiatry 2020;90:391-405.

[3] Felitti VJ, Anda RF, Nordenberg D, Williamson DF, Spitz AM, Edwards V, Koss MP, J S Marks JS. Relationship of childhood abuse and household dysfunction to many of the leading causes of death in adults: the adverse childhood experiences (ACE) study. Am J Prev Med 1998;14:245–58.

[4] Wolchik SA, Sandler IN. Handbook of children's coping with common life stressors. New York: Plenum, 1997.

[5] Nickerson A, Bryant RA, Aderka IM. The impacts of parental loss and adverse parenting on mental health: Findings from the national comorbidity survey-replication. Psychol Trauma 2013;5:119–27.

[6] Umberson D, Olson JS, Crosnoe R, Liu H, Pudrovska T, Donnelly R. Death of family members as an overlooked source of racial disadvantage in the United States. Proc Natl Acad Sci USA 2017;114:915–20.

[7] Hillis SD, Blenkinsop A, Villaveces, A, Annor FB, Liburd L, Massetti GM, Demissie Z, Mercy JA, Nelson III, CA, Cluver L, Flaxman S, Sherr L, Donnelly CA, Ratmann O, & Unwin, HJT. COVID-19–associated orphanhood and caregiver death in the United States. Pediatrics 2021;148:21-43.

[8] Currier JM, Neimeyer RA, Berman JS. The effectiveness of psychotherapeutic interventions for bereaved persons: A comprehensive quantitative review. Psychol Bull 2008;134:648–61.

[9] Sandler I, Gunn H, Mazza G, Tein JY, Wolchik S, Kim H, Ayers T, Porter M. Three perspectives on mental health problems of young adults and their parents at a 15-year follow-up of the family bereavement program. J Consult Clin Psychol 2018;86:845–55.

[10] Sandler I, Tein J-Y, Cham H. Long-term effects of the family bereavement program (FBP) on spousally-bereaved parents: grief, mental health, alcohol problems, and coping efficacy. Dev Psychopathol 2016;28:801–18.

[11] Anderson M, Jiang JJ. Teens, social media and technology 2018. Pew Research Center. URL: https://www.pewresearch.org/internet/2018/05/31/teens-social-media-technology-2018.

[12] Ziebland S, Wyke S. Health and illness in a connected world: How might sharing experiences on the internet affect people's health? Does sharing on the internet affect people's health? Milbank Q 2012;90:219–49.

[13] van Uden-Kraan CF, Drossaert CHC, Taal E, Shaw BR, Seydel ER, van de Laar MAFJ. Empowering processes and outcomes of participation in online support groups for patients with breast cancer, arthritis, or fibromyalgia. Qual Health Res 2008;18:405–17.

[14] Courtois CA, Gold SN. The need for inclusion of psychological trauma in the professional curriculum: A call to action. Psychol Trauma 2009;1:3.

[15] Ortiz R, Sibinga EM. The role of mindfulness in reducing the adverse effects of childhood stress and rrauma. Children (Basel) 2017;4:16.

[16] Lyon AR, Koerner K. User-centered design for psychosocial intervention development and implementation. Clin Psychol (New York) 2016;23:180–200.

[17] Lyon AR, Brewer SK, Areán PA. Leveraging human-centered design to implement modern psychological science: Return on an early investment. Am Psychol 2020;75:1067–79.

[18] Ayers TS, Wolchik SA, Sandler IN, Twohey JL, Weyer JL, Padgett-Jones S, Weiss L, Cole E, and Gary Kriege G. The family bereavement program: description of a theory-based prevention program for parentally-bereaved children and adolescents. Omega (Westport) 2013;68:293–314.

[19] Sandler IN, Ayers TS, Wolchik SA, Tein JY, Kwok OM, Haine RA, Twohey-Jacobs J, Suter J, Lin K, Padgett-Jones S, Weyer JL, Cole E, Kriege G, Griffin WA. The family bereavement program: efficacy evaluation of a theory-based prevention program for parentally bereaved children and adolescents. J Consult Clin Psychol 2003;71:587–600.

[20] Keng SL, Smoski MJ, Robins CJ. Effects of mindfulness on psychological health: a review of empirical studies. Clin Psychol Rev 2011;31:1041–56.

[21] Zhang Q, Wang Z, Wang X, Liu L, Zhang J, Zhou RL. The effects of different stages of mindfulness meditation training on emotion regulation. Front Hum Neurosci 2019;13:208.

[22] Chinoda S, Mutsinze A, Simms V, Chauke RB, Verhey R, Robinson J, Barker T, Mugurungi O, Apollo T, Munetsi E, Sithole D, Weiss HA, Chibanda D and Nicola Willis N.. Effectiveness of a peer-led adolescent mental health intervention on HIV virological suppression and mental health in Zimbabwe: Protocol of a cluster-randomised trial. Glob Ment Health (Camb) 2020;7:e23.

[23] Stice E, Rohde P, Shaw H, Gau JM. Clinician-led, peer-led, and internet-delivered dissonance-based eating disorder prevention programs: Effectiveness of these delivery modalities through 4-year follow-up. J Consult Clin Psychol 2020;88:481–94.

[24] Patalay P, Annis J, Sharpe H, Newman R, Main D, Ragunathan T, Parkes M, Clarke K. A pre-post evaluation of OpenMinds: a sustainable, peer-led mental health

literacy programme in universities and secondary schools. Prev Sci 2017;18:995–1005.

[25] Sandler IN, Wolchik SA, Ayers TS, Tein JY, Luecken L. Family bereavement [rogram (FBP) approach to promoting resilience following the death of a parent. Fam Sci 2013;4:87-94.

Section two: Acknowledgments

Chapter 10

About the editors

I Leslie Rubin, MD, is originally from South Africa where he trained in pediatrics and emigrated to the United States in 1976. He is currently Associate Professor in the Department of Pediatrics at Morehouse School of Medicine, Adjunct Associate Professor, Department of Pediatrics, Emory University School of Medicine, Director of Break the Cycle Program at the Southeast Pediatric Environmental Health Unit at Emory University (PEHSU), President and Founder of Break the Cycle of Health Disparities Inc, and Medical Director of The Rubin Center for Autism and Developmental Pediatrics in Atlanta, Georgia. He has been involved in the health care of children and adults with intellectual and developmental disabilities since 1977. In 1989, he and Allen Crocker published the first textbook on medical care for children and adults with developmental disabilities with the second edition in 2006. Sadly, Allen Crocker passed away in 2011, but, in partnership with Joav Merrick and others published the 3rd edition: "Health care for people with intellectual and developmental disabilities across the lifespan" with Springer in 2016. He currently directs interdisciplinary clinical programs for children with autism, cerebral palsy and other developmental disabilities and consults to a variety of programs including the Emory University Neurodevelopmental Exposure Clinic (ENEC), an interdisciplinary, research-based program looking at the impact of prenatal exposures on child development and behavior in the context of the social and economic disadvantage and health disparities. Among his awards for various activities, he received the Robert E Cooke Lifetime Achievement Award from the AADMD in 2015 and the Autism Achievement Award in 2016 from the Annual Conference and Exposition of Georgia, and the F Edwards Rushton CATCH Award from the American Academy of Pediatric in 2018, and most recently, was named one of 50 Advocate Heroes over the 50 years of Exceptional Parent Magazine. He is actively involved in the American Academy of Pediatrics as the Chair of the Georgia Chapter Environmental Health Committee and District X CATCH Facilitator for the AAP. He was on the US Environmental Protection Agency Board of Scientific Counsellors focusing on Sustainable Healthy Communities from 2016-2022 and is now on the National Advisory Council for Children and Disasters. He is also the Chair of the National PEHSU Steering Committee and is on the Advisory Councils of HERCULES, the Human Exposome Research Center at Emory University; and on the National START Advisory Committee, based at the University of New Hampshire. In 2004 he founded the Break the Cycle program which addresses children's environmental health disparities by recruiting bright university students to develop creative projects that will Break the Cycle and then publish their papers in international journals and books on public health. To date there have been more than 150 students from the USA, Latin America and Africa. The program received the Children's Environmental Health Excellence Award from the EPA in 2016. Email: lrubi01@emory.edu

Joav Merrick, MD, MMedSci, DMSc, born and educated in Denmark is professor of pediatrics, Division of Pediatrics, Hadassah Hebrew University Medical Center, Mt Scopus Campus, Jerusalem, Israel and Kentucky Children's Hospital, University of Kentucky, Lexington, Kentucky United States and professor of public health at the Center for Healthy Development, School of Public Health, Georgia State University, Atlanta, United States, the former medical director of the Health Services, Division for Intellectual and Developmental Disabilities, Ministry of Social Affairs and Social Services, Jerusalem, the founder and director of the National Institute of Child Health and Human Development in Israel. Numerous publications in the field of pediatrics, child health and human development, rehabilitation, intellectual disability, disability, health, welfare, abuse, advocacy, quality of life and prevention. Received the Peter Sabroe Child Award for outstanding work on behalf of Danish Children in 1985 and the International LEGO-Prize ("The Children's Nobel Prize") for an extraordinary contribution towards improvement in child welfare and well-being in 1987. In 2017 appointed a Kentucky Colonel by the Commonwealth of Kentucky, the highest honor the governor can bestow to a person. Email: jmerrick@zahav.net.il.

Chapter 11

About the Break the Cycle of Health Disparities Inc

Break the Cycle of Health Disparities Inc. (BCHD) is a private, not-for-profit 501c3, non-governmental organization dedicated to exploring the social, economic and environmental determinants of health in the context of children's health disparities and to use this to promote health equity for all children.

BCHD collaborates with the Southeast PEHSU to produce the annual Break the Cycle of Children's Environmental Health Disparities Program (Break the Cycle). Break the Cycle is a multidisciplinary academic research and training program that focuses on raising awareness of children's environmental health disparities and cultivating future leaders among university students in the fields of medicine, nursing, public health, law, social work, education and other related disciplines.

Each year, Break the Cycle invites students from a diversity of colleges and universities to develop projects that will "break the cycle of children's environmental health disparities". Break the Cycle faculty guides and monitors the progress of the students towards compeltion of their projects. The students present their completed projects at a national conference and their work is published in international journals. Over the past 15 years Break the Cycle has engaged over 150 students from 50 different university departments in 12 states in the USA, as well as students from Latin America, Europe and Africa, that have resulted in the publication of 13 journal supplements. These sets of projects form the basis for this book series.

In 2016, Break the Cycle received a Children's Environmental Health Excellence Award from the US Environmental Protection Agency for the achievements of the program.

BCHD has expanded its areas of interest and practice to Break the Cycle of Autism Disparities, Break the Cycle of Climate Change for Vulnerable Children, Break the Cycle of Environmental Degradation, Break the Cycle of Children's Mental Health Disparities, and Break the Cycle of Health Disparities for Native Children.

Contact

I Leslie Rubin MD
Associate Professor, Department of Pediatrics, Morehouse School of Medicine
Adjuct Associate Profesor, Department of Pediatrics, Emory University School of Medicine
Director, Break the Cycle Program, Southeast Pediatric Environmental Health Specialty Unit, Emory University School of Medicine
President and Founder, Break the Cycle of Health Disparities Inc
Medical Director, The Rubin Center for Autism and Developmental Pediatrics
750 Hammond Drive, Building 1, Suite 100, Atlanta, GA 30328, United States
Email: lrubi01@emory.edu
Website: www.breakthecycleprogram.org
Website: www.therubincenterforautism.org

Chapter 12

About the Pediatric Environmental Health Specialty Units (PEHSU)

The Pediatric Environmental Health Specialty Units (PEHSU's) are an interconnected system of regional centers located throughout the United States that respond to questions from public health professionals, clinicians, policy makers, and the public about environmental health concerns related to children and reproductive age adults. After fifteen years of programmatic operations, collaborations, and a growing desire to protect the health of children and reproductive age adults from environmental hazards, the PEHSU Program has gained the attention and respect of the pediatric and reproductive environmental medical community and families at risk from exposure to environmental contaminants. The PEHSU programs have a critical role in supporting the mission of the Agency for Toxic Substances and Disease Registry (ATSDR) to prevent or mitigate the adverse human health effects and diminished quality of life that result from exposure to hazardous substances in the environment and the mission of the US Environmental Protection Agency (EPA) to protect human health and the environment. The PEHSUs provide a credible, academic, non-commercial source of health information and clinical expertise regarding environmental toxins and their effects on children and reproductive age adults.

ATSDR and EPA established the PEHSUs to increase the capacity of health care providers to identify and treat environmental-related health conditions, prevent exposure to children and reproductive age adults, and communicate health risks from environmental exposures. The PEHSU Network includes teams of medical specialists (pediatricians, medical toxicologists, epidemiologists, obstetricians, nurses, nurse practictioners, occupational and environmental health physicians), public health professionals, researchers, psychologists, and educators to provide consultations, trainings, referrals and clinical services to health care providers, governmental agencies and the general public on pediatric and reproductive environmental health. PEHSUs also engage communities and stakeholders in public outreach projects

The National PEHSU Network helps individuals and communities to make informed decisions regarding environmental health concerns. Common concerns include lead poisoning, fungus or mold, mercury, pesticides, phthalates, air quality and school safety. There have also been national responses generated for hazards from wildfires, hurricanes, oil spills, carbon monoxide, mercury spills, de-icer leaks at airports, and industrial pollution.

While Poison Control Centers respond to acute toxic exposures, the PEHSU Network has expertise in long term, chronic low dose exposures, group exposures, and the development and dissemination of public messages. The PEHSU Network partners closely with local, state, and federal agencies and non-profit professional organizations in carrying out this work.

The PEHSUs collaborate with ATSDR and EPA to develop fact sheets targeting clinicians and the public on issues associated with flooding, hurricanes, wildfires, oil spills, formaldehyde, carbon monoxide poisoning, arsenic in foods, medical management of lead exposure, phthalates and bisphenl A, melamine, and other issues. They edit academic textbooks, publish manuscripts, and conduct outreach and educational programs to enhance pediatric and reproductive environmental health literacy.

The PEHSU's provide information online (website: www.pehsu.net) with a variety of materials to educate professionals and the general public in reproductive and children's environmental health through conferences, presentations and social media . PEHSU members serve on national boards and committees to advance collaborative activities and community expertise in environmental health. The PEHSUs train and mentor medical, toxicology, nursing, and other graduate students and provide hands-on opportunities in pediatric environmental medicine and reproductive epidemiology. The PEHSUs have advised first responders, parents, health officials, and school administrators on how to assess and mitigate environmental emergencies and address health-related findings. They have also provided training to establish PEHSUs in Chile, Argentina, Canada, Mexico, Vietnam, and Israel.

The PEHSUs serve to translate research findings into clinical and public health practice. PEHSU faculty are prepared to recognize, treat, and prevent toxic environmental exposures in children and communicate risk, treatment, and prevention strategies in a meaningful and culturally appropriate way.

Southeast PEHSU

The Southeast PEHSU, within the National PEHSU network, serves the southeastern United States and includes Alabama, North Carolina, South Carolina, Florida, Georgia, Kentucky, Mississippi and Tennessee. The Southeast PEHSU is based in the Nell Hodgson Woodruff School of Nursing at Emory University in Atlanta, GA and works closely with Region 4 of the US Environmental Protection Agency (EPA) and the Agency for Toxic Substances and Disease Registry (ATSDR) at the Centers for Disease Control and Prevention (CDC). The team includes Abby Mutic PhD, MSN, CNM (Assistant Professor and Certified Nurse Midwife), Leslie Rubin, MD (Developmental Pediatrician), Melissa Gittinger, DO (Medical Toxicologist), Rebecca Philipsborn, MD, MPA (Pediatrician), Victoria Green, MD, JD, MBA (Obstetrician Gynecologist), Claire Coles, PhD (Clinical Psychologist), Nathan Mutic, MS, MAT, MEd (Educator and Program Administrator), and Wayne Garfinkel, BSCE (formerly of Region 4 EPA). In addition, Benjamin Gitterman, MD (Pediatrician) works with the Southeast PEHSU on the Break the Cycle program.

Contact Southeast PEHSU

Abby Mutic, PhD, MSN, CNM
Director, Southeast Pediatric Environmental Health Specialty Unit
Nell Hodgson Woodruff School of Nursing, Emory University
1520 Clifton Road, Atlanta, GA 30322, United States.
Toll free tel: (877) 33 PEHSU or (877) 337-3478
Tel: (404) 727-7980
E-mail: sepehsu@emory.edu
Website: https://www.nursing.emory.edu/pages/southeastern-pediatric-environmental-health-specialty-unit

Chapter 13

About the National Institute of Child Health and Human Development in Israel

The National Institute of Child Health and Human Development (NICHD) in Israel was established in 1998 as a virtual institute under the auspices of the Medical Director, Ministry of Social Affairs and Social Services in order to function as the research arm for the Office of the Medical Director. In 1998 the National Council for Child Health and Pediatrics, Ministry of Health and in 1999 the Director General and Deputy Director General of the Ministry of Health endorsed the establishment of the NICHD.

Mission

The mission of a National Institute for Child Health and Human Development in Israel is to provide an academic focal point for the scholarly interdisciplinary study of child life, health, public health, welfare, disability, rehabilitation, intellectual disability and related aspects of human development. This mission includes research, teaching, clinical work, information and public service activities in the field of child health and human development.

Service and academic activities

Over the years many activities became focused in the south of Israel due to collaboration with various professionals at the Faculty of Health Sciences (FOHS) at the Ben Gurion University of the Negev (BGU). Since 2000 an affiliation with the Zusman Child Development Center at the Pediatric Division of Soroka University Medical Center has resulted in collaboration around the establishment of the Down Syndrome Clinic at that center. In 2002 a full course on "Disability" was established at the Recanati School for Allied Professions in the Community, FOHS, BGU and in 2005 collaboration was started with the Primary Care Unit of the faculty and disability became part of the master of public health course on "Children and society". In the academic year 2005-2006 a one semester course on "Aging with disability" was started as part of the master of science program in gerontology in our collaboration with the Center for Multidisciplinary Research in Aging. In 2010 collaborations with the Division of Pediatrics, Hadassah Hebrew University Medical Center, Jerusalem, Israel around the National Down Syndrome Center and teaching students and residents about intellectual and developmental disabilities as part of their training at this campus.

Research activities

The affiliated staff have over the years published work from projects and research activities in this national and international collaboration. In the year 2000 the International Journal of Adolescent Medicine and Health and in 2005 the International Journal on Disability and Human Development of De Gruyter Publishing House (Berlin and New York) were affiliated with the National Institute of Child Health and Human Development. From 2008 also the International Journal of Child Health and Human Development (Nova Science, New York), the International Journal of Child and Adolescent Health (Nova Science) and the Journal of Pain Management (Nova Science) affiliated and from 2009 the International Public Health Journal (Nova Science) and Journal of Alternative Medicine Research (Nova Science). All peer-reviewed international journals.

National collaborations

Nationally the NICHD works in collaboration with the Faculty of Health Sciences, Ben Gurion University of the Negev; Department of Physical Therapy, Sackler School of Medicine, Tel Aviv University; Autism Center, Assaf HaRofeh Medical Center; National Rett and PKU Centers at Chaim Sheba Medical Center, Tel HaShomer; Department of Physiotherapy, Haifa University; Department of Education, Bar Ilan University, Ramat Gan, Faculty of Social Sciences and Health Sciences; College of Judea and Samaria in Ariel and in 2011 affiliation with Center for Pediatric Chronic Diseases and

National Center for Down Syndrome, Department of Pediatrics, Hadassah Hebrew University Medical Center, Mount Scopus Campus, Jerusalem.

International collaborations

Internationally with the Department of Disability and Human Development, College of Applied Health Sciences, University of Illinois at Chicago; Strong Center for Developmental Disabilities, Golisano Children's Hospital at Strong, University of Rochester School of Medicine and Dentistry, New York; Centre on Intellectual Disabilities, University of Albany, New York; Centre for Chronic Disease Prevention and Control, Health Canada, Ottawa; Chandler Medical Center and Children's Hospital, Kentucky Children's Hospital, Section of Adolescent Medicine, University of Kentucky, Lexington; Chronic Disease Prevention and Control Research Center, Baylor College of Medicine, Houston, Texas; Division of Neuroscience, Department of Psychiatry, Columbia University, New York; Institute for the Study of Disadvantage and Disability, Atlanta; Center for Autism and Related Disorders, Department Psychiatry, Children's Hospital Boston, Boston; Department of Pediatric and Adolescent Medicine, Western Michigan University Homer Stryker MD School of Medicine, Kalamazoo, Michigan, United States; Department of Paediatrics, Child Health and Adolescent Medicine, Children's Hospital at Westmead, Westmead, Australia; International Centre for the Study of Occupational and Mental Health, Düsseldorf, Germany; Centre for Advanced Studies in Nursing, Department of General Practice and Primary Care, University of Aberdeen, Aberdeen, United Kingdom; Quality of Life Research Center, Copenhagen, Denmark; Nordic School of Public Health, Gottenburg, Sweden, Scandinavian Institute of Quality of Working Life, Oslo, Norway; The Department of Applied Social Sciences (APSS) of The Hong Kong Polytechnic University Hong Kong.

Targets

Our focus is on research, international collaborations, clinical work, teaching and policy in health, disability and human development and to establish the NICHD as a permanent institute in Israel in order to conduct model research and provide policy aspects in the field of interest.

Contact

Professor Joav Merrick, MD, MMedSci, DMSc
Director, National Institute of Child Health and Human Development, Jerusalem, Israel. E-mail: jmerrick@zahav.net.il

Section three: Index

Index

R

S

T

U

W